About The Author

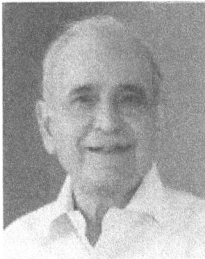

Dr Anil Gandhi was born in 1939. He completed his M.B.B.S in 1963 and started practicing as a family physician. He did his M.S in 1971 and for two decades from 1966 to 1986 was involved in providing healthcare including surgery in the rural areas of the Pune district. During this period he set up his own hospital in 1970 and did a lot of work for the middle class and also for economically backward classes. He has also acquired a diploma in colo-rectal surgery from St. Mark'sHospital, London in 1974 and read scientific papers in many conferences in India and abroad.

He was a teacher for some time at the B.J Medical College. Other colleges where he has taught are Tilak Ayurveda College, Bhartiyavidyapeeth and D.S Hom. Medical College in Pune. On the social front he was the founder chairman of a trust working for the tribal community. Ho was invited for a lecture at 'Vasant Vyakhyanmala' at Pune and Wai.

His Literary works include:

a) Mana Sarjana(his autobiography written in 2010, translated in Gujarati , Hindi and later in English)

b) Dhanwantari Gharoghari(about Health,2011)(Marathi)

c) Vicharimana(on social problems,2013). (Marathi)

d) Shodha Mancha(short stories, 2013).(Marathi)

e) High Tech Lifeline- on High Tech modalities of Health in English and Marathi)

f) Wrote a column in 'Sagun-Nirgun' in Maharashtra Times for 3 months.

g) He has also written on abstract subjects in 'Loksatta'.

BRAIN
THE
MASTERMIND

Dr. Anil Gandhi

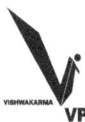

Vishwakarma Publications

BRAIN THE MASTERMIND

First Edition: November 2014
© Dr. Anil Gandhi
Mobile : 094 22 00 44 66
Email : ganilgulab@gmail.com

Published by:
Vishwakarma Publications
283, Budhwar Peth, Near City Post,
Pune - 411 002.
Phone : 020 20261157
Email : info@vpindia.co.in
Website : www.vpindia.co.in

Cover Design Credits
Meghnad Deodhar,
Vishwakarma Publications

Typeset and Layout
Vishwakarma Publications

Printed by
Repro India Limited, Mumbai

ISBN 978-93-83572-46-5

Dedication

Continuous research in all fields of science has contributed to the comfort and lifestyle of the human race. Neuroscientists are working hard to decode the many secrets of the brain. Perceptions learning memory emotions intelligence and cognition all are being extensively researched into.

Computer Scientists are decoding brain waves to extract information received and stored by the subject. They are trying to emulate the neural networks of the brain. They are trying their best to produce an intelligent machine. They also want to inculcate the cognitive abilities in the machines. It is possible that in a foreseeable future they will succeed.

I salute the scientific community and dedicate this book to their unflinching efforts.

Discerning Readers' Views

"Scientists are exploring the universe. The more they explore the more astounding and complex it becomes. The Oceanographers are making attempts to reach the bottom of the ocean. As they go deeper they realize how little they know. The Geo-scientists are also trying to reach the ultimate depths of our earth. Jules Verne the original and well known science fiction writer of the mid-nineteenth century described when none of the scientific explorations had begun the adventures of fictionalexplorers with imagination that was sheerly fantastic.in his famous books 20000 leagues Under the SeaandThe Journey to the Center of Earth. That was literary fantasy.(Jules Verne the well known science fiction writer of the mid-ninteenth century described with fantastic imagination the adventures of fictional explorers in novels like 20000 leagues Under the Sea).

In that same century philosophers psychologists and physiologists had begun an equally fantastic voyage to analyse and study the mind. The explorations of mind are proving to be more mysterious more difficult and far more challenging. The first and obvious question which continues to haunt them even today is "Where is this mind anyway?" It was common for people and poets to use the expression "My heart says that I love you" or many such things. Then all of us go through the so- called Hamlet's dilemma "to be or not to be " in which"one mind " says one thing and the " other mind " says exactly the opposite Are there two minds? In fact sometimes not only two but several minds give multiple options to you and you choose one, thinking that it is the right one. Is there only one mind with multiple expressions or many minds? And what do we mean by "My Mind"?

Where does the mind go when the body ceases to be? When does life finally end? Does mind continue to exist in the "soul"? Nobody has seen the soul. But then nobody has seen the mind either. However today most neurologists, psychologists, and even philosophers seem to agree that the mind is located in the brain. Of course a few scientists say that the mind is in the entire physiological structure; the nervous system blood veins muscles bones etc. but even they concede that the epicenter of all mental activity is the brain.

The explorations of the brain are the fascinating adventures undertaken by scientists. But how much do they really know as of today? Almost every day somewhere in the world's laboratories or in the neurologists' investigations of the brains of living people as well as those of dead scientists are trying to unravel the mystery. Whatever they have explored or understood is so "mind blowing" that it takes us on a wonderful journey of the sphere of knowledge.

Dr. Anil Gandhi's book provides us glimpses of all that is going on the world over in this truly exciting narrative. How do we think how do we remember or how do we forget? How do we laugh or cry? How do we interact with other people or with nature? How do we hate fight or attack? How do we learn? These are all attributes of our brain (or rather mind).

This book will enlighten the reader and make him more curious. In fact he will ask more questions and seek more (and even different) answers. But to make us more inquisitive it is necessary that our mind is provoked challenged and intrigued. Dr Gandhi's book will make us creatively uncomfortable in the sense that it will evict us out of the "comfort zones" in which we exist lazily. So read this book to enjoy this voyage of comfortable discomfort!"

Kumar Ketkar

"Believe it or not even at the age of 16 the human organ that attracted me most was the BRAIN. Even now it continues to be so most happily. Why and how so? Dr. Anil Gandhi's book Brain the Mastermind explains it. In a way it is a scary compendium of all kinds of ups and downs in and of the Brain. Discerning readers will find it enlightening."

Avinash Dharmadhikari

"A great spiritual master of the past hit the ground stoutly with his staff and shouted at his disciple "Byjeed are you there? Politely the follower replied ""Yes Master I'm here. A simple story but studded with many intriguing facets like who was Byjeed how did he know he was the one what is awareness how does it differ from consciousness where do both of them reside? In the brain or in the mind? What is either of them? Is the mind really there at all? How do both function and what is their structure? How do we think remember or forget? Or simply how do we stay awake or asleep? Why do we yawn snore or sneeze? Some people are clever and others are idiot. What do these terms imply? What are the diseases of the brain that we often hear about e.g. paralysis, dementia? Does the brain live as a whole or a part of it dies? And if it dies is life possible with a dead brain?

Interesting questions indeed! Answers to all such queries would be found in the book Brain the Master Mindwritten by a famous successful and senior surgeon of Pune Dr. Anil Gandhi. He has many books to his credit which are well received by readers.

The book easily engages attention of readers and makes a passionate reading. It is a "must for any reader with curiosity."

Dr. Ulhas Luktuke (Psychiatrist)

"Feeling thinking speech and action are the main criteria to study functions of the mind. These are all a result of the coordinated functioning of our brain starting from vital functions like locomotion breathing digestion and circulation. Brain controls all higher functions like reproduction ego hearing vision and all the functions of our mind. Mind therefore is a part of the various functions of our brain. Different parts of our brain control different functions.But the brain and the mind function as one unit as one organ of our body. Each part while performing the work allotted to it also has an influence on theother parts. Therefore the parts responsible for the functioning of the mind also have an impact on the parts controlling the body. Mind influences the body and the body influences the mind. Body-mind are viewed as one unit. If one wishes to understand the function of our body we must understand the mind. To understand the mind we must understand the working of our brain the seat of the mind. In this book Brain the Mastermind Dr. Anil Gandhi has done a remarkable job in explaining the working of the Brain as well as that of the mind. This working of the brain and the mind includes their structure functions and disorders so that the common man understands the terms used in the medical jargon."

Dr. H. V. Sardesai

"Dr Anil Gandhi a leading medical expert in Pune has written a very good book related to brain and its functioning. Titled "Brain : The Mastermind".

Most of us have very little knowledge of how exactly brain works. In fact many experts have still not figured out the answer. There are many beliefs and theories about it and some have become legends. Some spiritual gurus/orators have disseminated lot of information which is interpreted as divine knowledge. There is a need to look at this subject through a neutral and scientific lens.

I really appreciate the efforts taken by Dr Anil Gandhi to present a scientific view on this complex subject. Many interesting aspects such as Anatomy, Memory, Diseases and treatment awareness are covered in the book. The last chapter on 'Science and Religion' meeting is very interesting.

I appeal to the author Dr Gandhi to promote this book in many forums and translate in regional languages for widespread knowledge dissemination.

All the Best!"

Dr Deepak Shikarpur

"Dr. Anil Gandhi has come out with yet another masterpiece. This time it is about the brain. The title of the book Brain - the Mastermind itself is attractive as it explains the relationship between the brain and the mind.

The book explains the technology behind EEG ECOG and DCES and Brain Spyware etc. The chapter on the history and evolution of the brain and nervous system is very interesting indeed! It explains how the human brain developed through the process of natural selection.

The book explains the brain in a very simple manner. It describes in detail a number of exercises and diets that will help maintain the health of the brain.

This book is about the brain as much as about the mind and technology. Therefore you will find discussion on a variety of subjects such as virtual reality, intuition, lucid, dreams, memory, learning, artificial, intelligence, emotions, maturity and creativity, alertness, drugs, hypnosis, hallucinations, prejudices, delusions, religion, pain, paralysis, vertigo, spondylosis, yawning, sneezing, epilepsy, phobia, OCD, sleep, insomnia, moods, depression, sexual, dysfunctions, addictions, suicidal, instincts, neuro, toxins, Alzheimers, Dementias, Parkinsons, Disease, Psychosomatic, disorder, HIV and AIDS, headaches, Meningitis, Encephalitis, Thrombosis, tumours, near death experience, computational, psychology etc. The book also talks about the evolution and history of religion including topics like Moksha etc.

Dr. Anil Gandhi has explained all these concepts in a lucid and simple language making the book easy to understand even for a layperson. I congratulate Dr. Anil Gandhi for his efforts and wish him the best for all his future projects. I would recommend this book to not just students, housewives or teachers but just about anybody with an interest in this subject. A reader will certainly find himself or herself much more rich and better informed after reading this excellent book."

Achyut Godbole

Foreword

Human beings have an inherent curiosity about things in and around them. It has led to the unfolding of innumerable mysteries in nature which we call innovations. This inquisitiveness about their own bodies led to the dissection of dead bodies in the 14th century. In fact the first dissections were done by Maharshi Sushrut in India.He is regarded as the father of surgery. This was the first step in the study of human amatomy. Yet for a long time nobody made any attempt to peep inside the skull by breaking open the Cranium...The Heart was considered the source of all human emotions and thinking. The importance of the brain was realised much later. Cutting open the body in order to providerelief from pain was done initially by the clerics and the barbers for almost five to six centuries. Surgery as an art andscience got universal recognition only in 1743 in the UK. X-rays as diagnostic tools were developed in the late 19th century and the C.T in the late 20th century- Diagnosis of brain diseases and surgery of the brain took wings after this in the real sense. The idea of the modern computer was first conceived by Alan Turing (1946). Computer science has grown by leaps and bounds since then. In fact all ofthe scientific innovations including the computer are the creations of the human brain. Of late the scientists have been able to build super computers with neural networks similar to those of then eurons present in the brain. Modern day computers have beaten the human brain in speed, strength, non-fatigability and tenacity. The robots which are run and controlled by by computers can work in adverse circumstances like high temperature, extreme atmospheric conditions, pressures of the deep sea bed and harmful radiations. Even so computers cannot beat the human brain in emotions logical decision making, and all the functions of cognition as of today. Efforts are on to build intelligent if not cognitive machines. This has met with a fair amount of success. Computer scientists and neuroscientists from different disciplines are working together in this field of artificial intelligence. In fact they are together trying to reverse engineer the brain!

As a computer scientist I have a lot of curiosity about the amazing abilities of the human brain. My basic discipline is engineering. At times I feel I should have studied biology as well. I am of the opinion that the curriculum of engineering should include biology as one of the subjects. I am quite insistent on being a mentor in biology, and am trying to convince IIT Delhi and Engineering Colleges to include it in their curriculum. An integrated knowledge of the brain biology and computer science will be very handy for designing a computer with cognitive abilities.

When I read the book "Brain - the Mastermind" I thought that somebody was trying to satisfy at least partially my cherished desire to write a book on this subject. Dr Anil Gandhi has dared to write on a difficult subject of tremendous curiosity for a common man. He has really succeeded in explaining the technical terms in simple English.

The book starts with the sensational topic of "brain hacking" attracting the attention of the reader at once. Well begun is half done! He then covers the topics of interest to the researcher; right from the structure and functions of the brain evolution of the nervous system and the development of the brain in the most primitive living beings to the most evolved man. The development of the brain in the human embryo, and modern tools useful for research on the brain have also been explained.

The second part stimulates an interesting discussion of the all-pervasive mind. Light is thrown on the faculties of the mind along with all its facets - like, learning, memory, skills and talents.

The next part starts with "pain". Nature has given us nothing unnecessarily not even "pain".

The example of a boy born without the sensation of pain is quite interesting. He concludes "Pain is a friend. A friend in need is a friend indeed!" Vascular accidents of the brain leading to strokes are discussed. Nobody likes to be handicapped and helpless. Measures which can help avoid them to the possible extent are suggested.

The last two chapters on the evolution of religions and the concepts of moksha, mukti, videhmuki and transcendence are quite interesting. The scientific discussion on the transcendental feelings of people near death experiences (NDE) the experiments on a Tibetan Monk with the help of functional MRI while practicing transcendental meditation (TM) have been cited to throw light on both religion and science bringing them together.

I sincerely congratulate Dr Anil Gandhi for coming out with such an informative and educative book on a subject at the heart of every common man in a language which can be assimilated by a common reader.

I am sure every human brain would like to be enlightened on the subject of the human brain.Everybody should read and keep this book in his personal library since it is the newest frontier of research and scientific exploration.

Dr. Vijay Bhatkar

Preface

I have been learning all the time. I have read some extraordinarily informative books on the subject. The most fascinating books I came across on the subject were 'Making the Most of Your Brain' compiled by the Readers Digest and Dr. Vilayanur S. Ramachandran's book 'The Emerging Mind' published by BBC. Another book which I found very informative is 'Karta Karavita' written in Marathi by Panase, Kshirsagar and Deshmukh. Surfing the internet yields a large treasure of knowledge on all subjects and the brain is no exception.

I am aware of the vastness of the subject which cannot be covered even within hundreds of treatises. In this small book about the brain it is proposed to explain a few interesting facts about the evolution structure and working of this phenomenal brain from the medical point of view.

The core message or the very purpose of the book is to make people aware of the simple measures to prevent birth defects of the brain and the nervous system.

Please refer to the images after page no. 80 and prevention of these deformities on Page no. 86. There is good news that The Awareness Campaign for Prevention of Spina bifida, anencephaly and Hydrocephalus

[NTDs] with Periconceptional Folic Acid supplement is being run by Jain Doctors Federation and Spina bifida Foundation. This is as good as a blessing.

Electronic media and the internet have opened a magic box of knowledge on any and every subject. So it was thought that the era of newspapers periodicals and books may end now. At least as of today the print media exists in the form of newspapers and periodicals. Books still retain a position in the heart of an avid reader.. After the success of my book High Tech Life Line written with an intention of adding to the General Knowledge of the common reader regarding medical concepts, I felt a compulsion to write about the brain and the nervous system. It gives me great pleasure in presenting to you, BRAIN - THE MASTER MIND.

Acknowledgments

Dr. H. V. Sardesai and Dr. Ulhas Luktuke have given me useful suggestions in preparing this book. Eminent computer-scientist Dr. Vijay Bhatkar has been very gracious to write the foreword. Eminent personalities like Kumar, Ketkar Achyut Godbole, Avinash Dharmadhikari, Dr. Deepak Shikarpur, Dr. H. V. Sardesai and Dr. Ulhas Luktuke have been very kind in writing previews. Dr. Supriya Sahasrabuddhe has done an excellent job of editing. Dr. Prakash Doke has been very kind and has provided me with all important photographs of specimens of the brain. Ajit Dharmadhikari has taken pains to make all the illustrations presentable. I am grateful to Dr. Ravindra Vora and Dr. Sudhakar Jadhav from Pediatric Surgery Centre and P. G. Institute Sangli for sending photographs of congenital anomalies of the brain for printing in this book. Logistic support of my family members and especially of Parth Gandhi and Ritu Shah was very encouraging.

I thank Bharat Agarwal of Vishwakarma Publications, due to whom this book has seen the light of day. I also thank Parag Joshi for the fine D T P work. I cannot resist but thank Dr. K. H. Sancheti who is an all - weather friend to me for everything that I do.

Contents

If wishes were Horses...

As a student I had learnt a proverb, 'If wishes were horses, beggars would ride them.'

The truth has changed. Even beggars will now aspire for something modern. In everyone's life most of the things have changed. This credit goes to the phenomenal progress in science and technology. Physically and mentally handicapped people were very unfortunate in the past. Things have changed for them as well. The problems of brain, nerves and muscles confineded the unfortunate victims to bed or a wheel chair. They could not dream of doing anything worthwhile to improve their own life. They could not think of doing some useful work for others. There is a sea change now. Take the glaring example of Stephen Hawking. He is confined to a wheel chair. Cannot move his legs, arms and hands, he can wink his eyelids. His brain and thought processes are very sharp. He uses the thought process and movement of his eyelids as the virtual hand (mouse) on the computer. With all the handicaps he is able to use the computer for research in mathematics, physics and cosmology. He is the Director of a research centre at the University of Cambridge.

I think it is time to change the proverb if wishes were horses the beggars would ride. Shall we now say 'You can ride on your wishes and rule the world!'

1 Hacking The Brain

"What a piece of work is man!

How noble in reason, how infinite in faculty!"

Shakespeare's Hamlet said this in the seventeenth century with a sense of wonder in an age when science had just started to progress. Much scientific research has gone into the working of the human body within the last four centuries and still the sense of wonder has not diminished because the human body is a fantastic machine which has not been explored fully even today. It is the first fact of human existence. There is a purpose behind the design and functioning of all the organ systems in the body. When the brain is dead it is the end of all the organs and systems unless they are kept alive for a limited time by the recent technological gadgets. The human body and especially the brain in it are tremendous forces that have been continuously amazing mankind since ages. Scientists, thinkers, poets, yogis, and scholars of every science have been trying to understand the working of the brain fully.

Every cell has a precise structure and function. Though every part of this machine is important the most important and vital of all is the master controller the brain.

The importance of the vital roles of the heart and lungs was recognized by people long ago. The roles of the kidneys and liver were also understood later but the role played by the brain in controlling these vital organs and every other organ, systems and cells was recognized much later than that. Now we know that the brain is the head of the institution. It is the conductor of the orchestra known as the human body. The precise structure of each organ or cell the fine tuning of the functions of each cell, each organ and system in the body owes its control to the brain. Not only these overtly visible structures and functions, but even the invisibles like learning memory, experience, emotions, intelligence the evolutionary instincts of self protection and propagation of the DNA are controlled by the master controller - the brain.

The progress of science has brought some evils and one among them is the hacking of this great master controller the brain. Modern means of communication have given us many comforts. They almost instantly provide a lot of facilities. They were thought to be a safe way of communication but unfortunately they are not. Service providers have a record of all the communication carried out through them. They can exploit such information for commercial purposes. When people became aware that their communication is not secret any longer there was a hue and cry as there was a danger to the privacy of individuals. When we talk or write, our views are not necessarily our honest thoughts. Relatives, friends and even the fiancée may

The conscious mind always censors the information or the thought which we want to express to the outer world. We may have a sinister thought in our mind but we express only niceties contrary to our thoughts for social acceptability.

have no inkling of what is really in our mind. There is no way they can peep in to our minds. All the real thoughts are a very closely guarded secret. Nobody else has access to them and others have no option but to trust the niceties enacted by us.

Curiosity and necessities are origins of invention. Man has been exploring almost all the fields of life. All the secrets of nature can be decoded one day. However, it took a long time to study the structure and functions of the human body. The structure and function of the human brain is still a big challenge. The thought process of the human brain is still an enigma to neuroscientists. Scientists are claiming only partial success in decoding of thoughts and memories as of now. The following are some methods of getting to know the working of the brain.

EEG (Electro-Encephalo Gramme)

The EEG is a recording of the action potentials of the brain on a graphic tracing. The ECG of similar action potentials of the heart is common knowledge as compared to the EEG. The EEG is done after applying multiple electrodes to the scalp and face. These electrodes pick up electrical signals from the neurons (brain cells) and plot them in a graphic form on a paper. This EEG was invented to study epileptic fits in patients to start with. Now it is also used for sleep studies, brain activity in coma and to diagnose brain tumors strokes and other brain disorders as an adjunct to C.T and MRI. It is also used for confirming brain death to support clinical judgment.

This is the history of EEG. In 1875, Richard Caton first recorded the electrical phenomena of the exposed brain belonging to a rabbit. In 1912 in Russia, Vladimir Neminsky published the first animal EEG. Hans Berger recorded the first human EEG in Germany in 1924. In 1934, Fisher and Lowenback demonstrated the abnormal epileptiform spikes in the EEG.

ECoG –

Electrocorticography – Neurosurgeons implant strips and grids of electrodes (or penetrating electrodes in depth) in the brain. The recording of brainwaves by directly applying the electrodes to the brain is termed as Electrocorticography.

DCES

Direct Cortical (brain) Electrical Stimulation mapping along with ECoG is a method used to study the brain function. A combination of various brain imaging techniques like functional MRI (fMRI) with EEG or ECoG have been used with advantage.

The same principle of recording and interpretation of brain waves is being used by neuroscientists to study the areas of the brain for various sensory and motor functions and also to study dreams. All such data is fed into a sophisticated computer. These super computers are now able, with experience, to reconstruct visual images, auditory signals taste, smell, signals, touch, temperature and pain and pressure signals. This is not all. Scientists are probing the information stored in the memory and the thought process of the brain. Thus, decoding these signals will enable the neuroscientists to peep into the mind, understand and record its secret thoughts though, nobody likes to divulge them.   .

Researchers are also contemplating deleting or changing the information stored by the brain in the memory. This will change the person's identity and behavior and be the cause of identity crisis in future.

In short like computers human brains might be vulnerable to hackers. Technology is already allowing scientists to read peoples thoughts and even plant new ones in the brain.

Philip Low is developing a portable brain – the iBrian. Freeman explains that people with some form of paralysis still have healthy brain activity. Using the brain they could use thoughts to control a virtual hand on a computer screen. The classic example is Stephen Hawking. Some neuroscientists are already translating the language of the brain into plain English. Gallant and his associates showed people different images while measuring their brain activity via functional MRI. From the brain activity Gallants team can reconstruct the approximate images people see. Scientists are also developing a dictionary of concepts that allows them to guess what people are thinking and about the images they are seeing. If thoughts could be decoded could they also be altered? What if other people could hack into a persons brain and plant new thoughts there?

Well known novelist George Orwell had already thought of this idea. His famous novel 1984 was written in 1948. He shows his heros brain hacked with a fear technique after which this hero starts adoring the same person who had been his enemy.

Brain Spyware -

Users of headgear devices can download third party applications. In case of EEG devices, access to the raw EEG signals could be unrestricted. A potential malicious attacker could write "Brain Spyware" (software) to harvest private information from the user which could be legitimately downloaded as an app.

Brain hacking is the act of reading the contents of the human brain and modifying it. Is technology mature enough to allow hackers to penetrate our mind? Brain hacking explores the possibility of attacking the human brain to extract sensitive information.

Thus the human brain may be vulnerable to hacking

attacks. Scientists used a commercial device off the shelf of the brain computer interface for brain hacking resulting in the disclosure of information that victims had in their minds. The brain computer interface consists of –

1) Hardware (EEG) equipped with a series of sensors placed directly on the human scalp.

2) Software designed to interpret brain activity signals – (decoding Brain waves)

The price of this brain computer interface is just $200-300.

Brain hacking is a reality with high reliability. It has to be practised with informed consent so that medical ethics are not violated. Presently there is no technology for brain hacking (neuro-hacking) in the absence of the persons consent and co-operation. It is thought that usable neuro-hacking of this type is still years away but if it happens it is dangerous because it will be another tool in the hands of terrorists.

Neuro Criminology

A time may come when we may be able to do brain scans to determine whether a defendant is guilty of premeditated murder or merely of manslaughter.

Tender feelings are not in the touch of receptors but in the interpretation of the sensory cortex of the brain. Melody is not in the voice or instruments but in the interpretation of the auditory cortex. Provoking scents are just air borne vapors of chemicals. It is the olfactory cortex that gives the meaning and pleasure of smell. Taste of food is not in the food but in the sensory cortex stimulated by the gustatory buds.

Hacking The Brain.

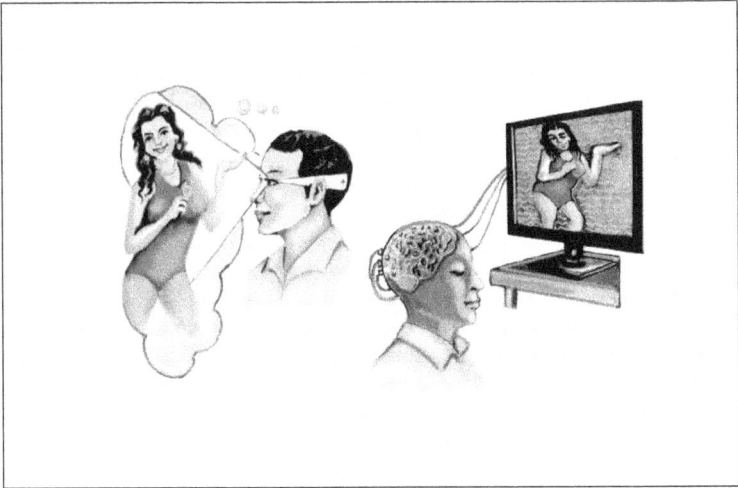

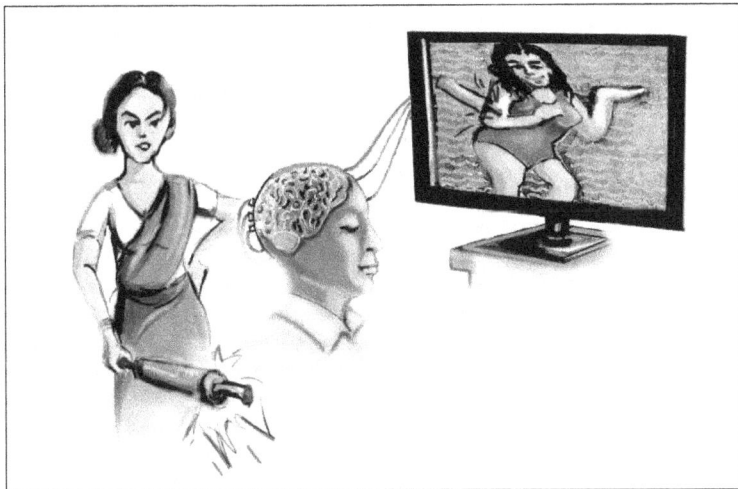

Brain Stem, Spinal Cord, Pineal Gland, Pituitary Gland

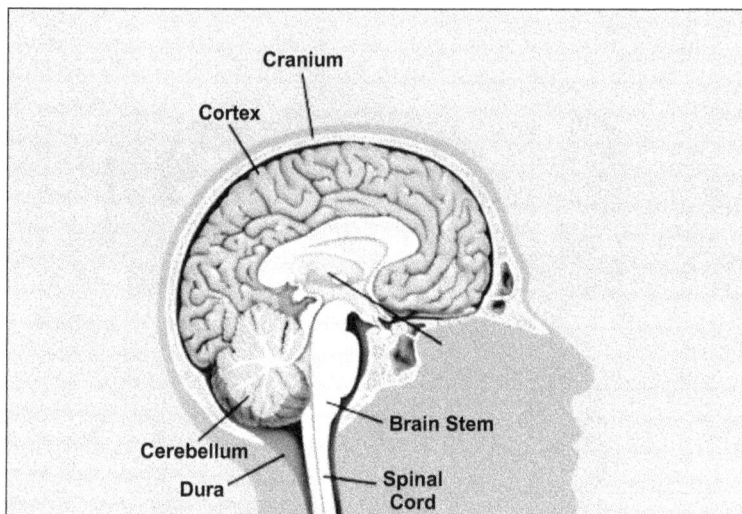

Cranium

Cortex

Brain Stem

Cerebellum

Dura

Spinal Cord

External Surface Lobes of Brain

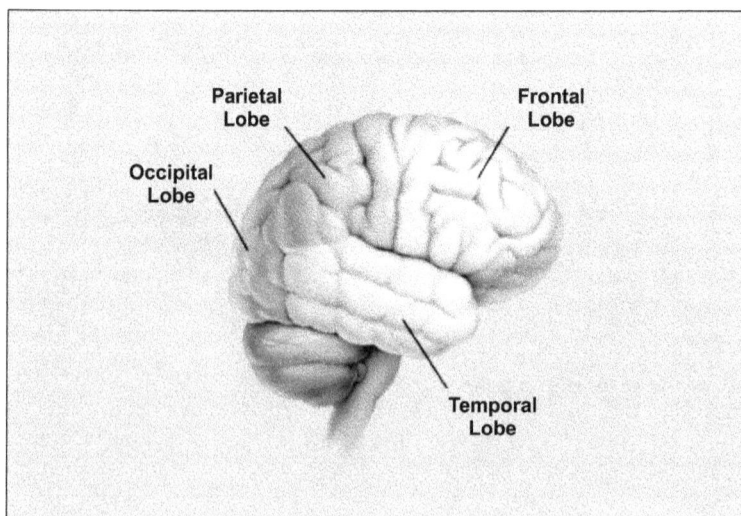

Parietal Lobe

Frontal Lobe

Occipital Lobe

Temporal Lobe

2 Evolution and History of The Brain

Just as animal and plant species have evolved, the brains and organs in animals have also evolved in order to adapt to the changes in the surroundings and the requirements dictated by the changed circumstances.

About thirty crore years ago the reptilian brain needed to control breathing, heart beats and balance of the body and also to help procurement of food by locomotion. This was done by the pons and medula. Twenty crore years back, acquisition of the skills of emotion, sexual instinct and fighting spirit became possible because of the acquisition of the hippocampus cerebellum and the limbic system. Ten crore years ago, the skills of language thinking and analysis were achieved on account of the development of the neo cortex. These changes increased the size of the brain. The size and shape of the skull changed to suit these changes in the size of the brain.

These ends are met by the microbes and plants though there is (nothing similar to the brain in them) but they do have chemical means for producing electrical potentials and they do exhibit abilities which respond to the environment. With evolution, animals started showing the presence of neurons and nerve fibers. In the process of evolution at the higher rung of the ladder,

The main function of the brain and the nervous system is to make the living being aware of its surroundings respond to it feed itself protect its own life and propagate its DNA.

large collections of neurons assumed the form of primitive brains. Human beings started with the brain weighing 350-400 gm in Australopithecus and progressed to the present 1400 gm brain in Homosapiens. The weight of an elephants brain is more than the human brain but if we consider the proportion of the weight of human brain and that of human body we see that human beings have larger brains than elephants.

Biologists and neuroscientists think that altruism evolved on the basis of kinship. The urge to bestow favors on family members has led to rapid development of the human brain. As the IQ and EQ of human beings developed and they achieved extraordinary skills in many ways, the cerebral hemispheres (Neo-Cortex) evolved more rapidly into the present form.

In the process of evolution, new capacities are added to the brain and older ones are also retained. The amygdala hippocampus and thalamus (parts of the primitive brain) are the main components of the limbic system that are retained for their function and newer functions of speech and skills are added.

The increase in the size of the brain was possible because of the increase in the number of neurons but the development of various higher faculties was achieved through increase in the number of synaptic connections between the neurons and the increase in glial cells. The glial cells act as a support system to the neurons. Prof. Stephen Qunon from Toronto University notes that human habitation in the ancient times took place near rivers and the seas. Sea food is very rich in Docosahexenoic Acid (DHA). DHA is very useful for the growth of nervous tissues. It is thought that this supplement brought about the rapid growth and evolution of the brain. The people staying away from the seas did not grow or evolve fast.

The changes that occurred during evolution were carried further in later generations by genes by the process of natural selection. They were improved upon further in the process of evolution in gen next.

However there are missing links in the theories of evolution in general. Survival and propagation are the primary evolutionary instincts of all the living beings. Be they viruses, bacteria, plants, insects, crawlers or the most evolved of them like human beings. All living beings need to understand favorable or unfavorable surroundings and need to respond appropriately in order to achieve the goals of self preservation and propagation. This is achieved by the signals coming in (received) and the signals sent out by the species. The signals may be chemical or electrical. Even electrical signals are created by the action potentials generated by the chemical reactions in the cells. These chemical or chemical-turned-electrical signals help the microbes to know the surroundings. If the environment is hostile, it makes them go into a shell for hibernation, stay in the dormant stage may be for hundreds of years only to come alive once the environment becomes friendly. As we go up the ladder of evolution we find the development of primitive nerve fibers and ganglion (collections of neurons). Ganglia are located at intervals of segments which take over this function of the two - way communication of chemically mediated electrical stimuli. At a higher step of evolution, these collections of neurons become more pronounced and we call them the brain. Usually, the brain is placed in the head end of the organism.

The brain is the great coordinator for all. So far the scientists have not been able to understand well defined structures like neurons or nerve fibers in plants. However, definite action potential in the form of electrical impulses can be demonstrated in carnivorous plants. The plant Venus Flytrap instantly traps insects that come close to its receptor hair. Attempts at recording electrical activity in the trap showed electrical potentials identical to the ones seen in the nerves of animals. The response of all the plants to sunlight is an established fact. They compete with each other for space to reach sunlight and in order to have nutrition below the ground via the roots. It is also interesting to note that the plants do not exhibit this competition with their kin i. e. plants of their own species. It is thought to be an altruistic trait of plants. Some scientists claim that plants have perception of pain and try to protect themselves from predators. They use thorns, smells and poisonous substances as their defense against predators and try to protect their own lives. All of us know the ingenious ways they use in the form of attractive shapes, colours, smell and nectar for attracting insects to help pollination and the resultant propagation.

> Intelligence is not the monopoly of the brain. From the bodies of humans, animals plants to the level of individual cells and unicellular organisms all exhibit intelligent behavior and precise and appropriate functions according to their needs.

Sir Jagdish Chandra Bose the eminent biologist invented a device called the Cerograph to see the effect of soft music on plants. He showed that plants exposed to music grew better than their peers that were not given musical therapy. A research by Michigan University has shown that some plants have a rudimentary nerve structure in place. They are capable of identifying danger signals and they communicate them to their peers. It is difficult to explain how they do that.

The microbes are too tiny to have a well defined nervous system. The hydra has a network of nerves the sea star has a nerve ring and radial fibers flat worms, leeches and insects have tiny brains and nerve cords.

At a higher level of evolution fish amphibians, reptiles and birds possess a well-developed brain and nervous system. Mammals have better defined brains with demonstrable divisions such as forebrain midbrain and hindbrain. Development of higher faculties of learning memory speech and emotions are a gift of the well-developed cerebral hemispheres in human beings. There seems to be a direct relation between the brain volume or weight and the higher faculties.

The brains of apes weigh around 300 to 350 gm. But that of the Javanese homoerectus is 930 gm Chinese homoerectus is 1029 gms but there is a quantum jump to 1350 gm of the Homo-sapiens or the present human race. In the process of evolution changes happened gradually and spread over millions of years. The big jump from apes to humans makes some scientists believe that the human race has not evolved from the apes. Some scientists have put the theories that the present human beings could be a genetically engineered species of ancient aliens. There are evidences of huge structures and awesome wonders like the pyramids all over the world where high tech knowledge and equipment must have been used. It was simply beyond the capacity of the primitive stone-age human beings on earth to do it. This gives credence to the theory that ancient aliens created the human race on the earth.

Intelligence and Artificial Intelligence (A. I.)

There is no single definition of intelligence. Plants and animals have limited intelligence. Normally logic, abstract thinking, understanding, self-awareness, communication, learning, emotions, memory, planning, creativity and problem solving skills together constitute intelligence. Human beings are blessed with unlimited intelligence. Individuals vary in their intellectual capacity. It is very difficult to evaluate intelligence quantitatively. At times the different skills have been classified as emotional social musical personal interpersonal and ecological intelligence. So far cognitive intelligence is considered an exclusive asset of human beings.

With advances in computing machines scientists have become confident that they will be able to produce machines with perfect intelligence soon. Alan Turing, a British mathematician pioneered the concept of computers in 1950. He was sure that it was possible to design an intelligent machine and the machine would become cognitive and alive in that sense, though not in the biological sense. Turing dreamt of it long back. In 2014 his dream has not come true but surely great progress has been made in that direction. Turing thought of testing machines for intelligence by questions and answers. This method is now called the "Turing Test. An international competition is held every year in which scientists working on Artificial Intelligence can participate. The best performer is honored with the Turing Prize.

John McCarthy was the first person to use the term Artificial Intelligence for the science of engineering engaged in making intelligent machines. Computer science, psychology, neuroscience and engineering are working together towards the aim of creating machines with Artificial Intelligence. Such an intelligent machine is expected to behave intelligently, learn and adapt to a particular situation and take logical decisions to suit the situation. In short, it should have its own mind to think and act.

At present machines are useful for automated tasks requiring intelligent behavior. They can control plan and schedule the production of items. These machines can answer medical, diagnostic and consumer questions. They have the ability to recognize the hand writing natural language speech and face of a person. These machines are also used for strategic games like chess and other videogames.

At present the human brain is the only machine of this sort if we can call it a machine.

Ray Kurgweil had built a computer as a high school student. He worked a lot on Artificial intelligence. He developed and sold reading machines for the blind, music synthesizers and speech recognition softwares. Kurgweil says that evolution of intelligence happens but it takes millions of years to effect change. The human brain works much faster. He feels that man can create a machine more intelligent than his own brain and his creations will surpass him. Here he presupposes that the human brain is a machine and that an alternative could be built. There are opposing views that properties such as consciousness and free will are unique to the human mind and are difficult to replicate. The present day machines have pattern recognition but no logical thinking capacity.

> We have not yet clearly understood the human mind. If the mind is only the sum total of the functions of the brain then it is possible to create a machine with a recognizable mind.

Robotics is extensively using A.I. technologies for vision pattern recognition, knowledge engineering, decision making and natural language understanding. The role of the robots using A. I. is not to displace human creativity but to amplify it. The A I machines may see translating telephones intelligent assistants at work or at home completely driverless cars or pilotless planes. It will be possible to identify the finger and voice prints with A. I.

Kurgweil says that even if A.I. replaces the whole industry there will be a net gain of jobs. Fields like communication teaching learning selling strategic decision making and innovation will continue to be done by human beings. Learning of children will be on portable computers running "intelligent and entertaining courseware. Papers examinations electronic mail and even 'love notes' will be sent on wireless networks. All the advanced power of A I will alter warfare. Laser and particle beams will be in action. Already there is a change in medicine- computer diagnosticians' coordinated data banks of patient histories, and realistic simulations for drug trials. Robotically assisted telesurgery has already entered the medical field.

This leaves humans free for research organization of knowledge banks administration and of course "comfort caring". Handicapped individuals are being greatly assisted by the advancing technology with reading machines hearing machines and robotic exoskeleton even today. The example of an A.I. machine helping a severely handicapped scientist Stephen Hawking is well known.

The machine (computer) may have a better speed than the brain but the brain always beats the machine in flexibility. Scientists are trying to make intelligent machines with consciousness but these are still out of reach. Nobody knows what the time frame for the future will be. Nor can the machine work on previous experience as of today.

Most of the things in everyone's life have changed today. This credit goes to the phenomenal progress of science and technology. Physically and mentally handicapped people were thought to be very unfortunate in the past. Things have changed for them as well. The problems of the brain, nerves and muscles confined the unfortunate victims to a bed or a wheel chair. They could not dream of doing anything worthwhile to improve their own life. They could not think of doing any useful work for others. There is a sea change now. Take the glaring example of Stephen Hawking. He is confined to a wheel chair and cannot move his legs arms and hands. He can only wink his eyelids. However his brain and thought processes are very sharp. He uses the thought processes and movement of the eyelids as the virtual hand (mouse) on the computer. With all the handicaps he is able to use the computer for research in mathematics, physics and cosmology. He is the Director of a Research Centre at the University of Cambridge

Neural networks

Artificial neural networks of computers give them an advantage over other computers. This has similarities to the networks of neurons in the human brain. The network is trained with examples. The network learns to make generalizations based on experience of the training data and can apply this knowledge when presented with inputs. This enables them to recognize speech or analyze financial trends. Still, it cannot match the capabilities of a human brain.

Mirror Neurons

An interesting observation was made. When a monkey grabs a peanut and another watches it, the set of similar neurons in both the monkeys are firing. These are both called mirror neurons. Stick your tongue out at a newborn baby and baby will stick its tongue out too.

In highly evolved human beings if one observes a sad mood or a jolly mood of the dear ones, similar mirror neurons fire together, and so the observing person also changes his mood. These mirror neurons may have played an important role in human evolution. One of the hallmarks of our species is what we call culture. Cultural transmission of information is what has characterized us humans.

3 Geography of The Brain

The intention of this book is to add to the general medical knowledge of the common man. Our knowledge about this master controller is of recent origin but we are trying to understand more and more every moment. We owe our recent knowledge to the continuous hard work of scientists. Yet we are far away from a complete understanding of the structure and functions of the brain. No human brain seems to be able to get full knowledge of the human brain. However this book cannot be a means of diagnosis of ailments. There is no alternative for family physicians and specialists in case of health problems.

Detailed information about the anatomy of the brain, the peripheral and the autonomic nervous system is beyond the scope of this book. The aim here is to acquaint the common readers with the gross anatomy so that they get an idea of the general functions of the brain. Hence let us get to know a little about the geography of the brain and the nervous system. It is the chief executive of the human body in general and the central

> The description of the structure or geography of the brain may be difficult but is useful to understand the elaborate functions and diseases of the brain.

nervous system in particular. It is formed of two large cerebral hemispheres separated from each other by a longitudinal (sagital sulcus) central fissure extending from the front to the back (antero-posterior). It is deep down to the corpus callosum. The corpus callosum is an aggregation of the nerve fibres coming from both of the cerebral hemispheres.

If we see the earth from outer space we do not find any dividing lines as in the maps. The artificial lines drawn by human beings have divided the globe into different parts called countries. Similarly there are no dividing lines between the various centers of the brain. They are man-made but in reality they merge into one another. If a particular sensory or motor organ stops functioning for some reason, or because of some congenital defect, the areas of the brain earmarked for that function are shrunk and are re-distributed for other functions with a view of compensating for the lost faculty. This is always seen in case of congenital blindness. The centers for hearing, smell and touch acquire more areas and try to compensate for the important visual function at least partially. Each cerebral hemisphere is further divided (artificially) in the frontal lobe in the front, the occipital lobe on the back side; the portion between these two is the parietal lobe. This lobe and small part of the frontal lobe sit on the temporal lobe. The brainstem consisting of the pons and medulla in the front and the cerebellum at the back, form the base on which the temporal lobe and the occipital lobe rest.

The arbitrary division of the brain is the right brain and the left brain. Both of them function together unless one is affected by trauma or disease.

The entire cerebral cortex shows elevations (the gyri) and depressions (sulci). This is nature's ingenious way of providing an extensive surface area for the cerebral cortex.

There are some prominent sulci. The one at the junction of the frontal and parietal lobes is called the central sulcus. It runs almost at a right angle to the central sulcus. The gyrus in front (anterior) of the central sulcus is called the pre central gyrus which houses the motor functions. The gyrus behind the central sulcus is called the post-central gyrus and it takes care of the somato-sensory functions. The largely developed cerebral cortex of human beings is also called neo-cortex. It is useful in higher faculties like language speech analytical abilities, skills, emotions and thinking which makes the human beings different from all other animals.

The limbic system is the oldest part of the brain on an evolutionary scale and lies deeply encompassed by the cerebral hemi-spheres. The limbic system is formed by the thalamus hippocampus, the amygdala and hypothalamus. The limbic system reacts to stimuli such as thirst and activities related to self–protection such as responding to danger signals. It also plays an important part in the expression of emotions. The brain stem lies beneath the limbic system. The all important vital functions of breathing, heartbeats, blood pressure and temperature regulation are the prime duties of the brain stem. The brain stem stimulates emotions. It is also responsible for attention and consciousness. The cerebellum or small brain is attached to the back of the brain stem. It mainly controls movements, co-ordination, and balance of the body and movements of eyes.

The brain does not fully develop during foetal life but a couple of years after birth. The surface of the cerebral cortex shows hardly any gyri and sulci. Perhaps that is not the need of the hour. The foetus is not exposed to the outside world. It is in the safe custody of the mother. All the requirements of life are available to it without any effort whatsoever. If all these functions were to be done by the foetal brain it would need to grow and such a growth would be harmful to the baby and the mother during child birth. To suit all these functions, when the foetus is in the womb of the mother, the brain is comparatively small in order to facilitate the journey to the outer world through the narrow birth passage. In addition to this the skull bones are separate pieces with gaps (fontanallae) and un-united suture joints between them. This not only facilitates easy delivery with the moulding but also provides room for rapid growth of the brain within the first two years of life after birth. The joints and fontanallae are closed only after this objective is achieved.

The first two years of life are very crucial for a human being. This period leads to concurrent fast development of the structure and functions of the brain and the nervous system. This rapid growth with limited space available for expansion gives rise to numerous folds on the surface of the brain which is comparatively very smooth at birth. This surface looks gray in colour and hence is called gray matter. Bodies of neurons are located in the gray matter. The fibers extending from these neurons which have a length of a millimeter to a meter lie deeper in the gray matter and look white. This is known as white matter.

There are more than a hundred billion neurons in the brain. These cells have very fine projecting fibers. The shorter ones (dendrons) receive signals from other cells while the longer ones carry signals to other cells (Axons). The zone of transition between the axons and the dendrons are called synapses or synaptic connections. The transmission of the electrical impulses from and to the neurons via these synapses is achieved with a chemical substance known as the neurotransmitter.

There are about one to ten thousand connections for every single neuron. Neurons vary in size from 4 microns to 100 microns. There are supporting cells in between the neurons called glial cells. Persons like Einstein or Lenin were outstanding geniuses. Scientists have been trying for some time to check if the brain of a genius and that of an ordinary man is different either grossly or microscopically. They did not find any big difference. However recently they have discovered that the brain of Einstein had larger number of glial cells. The glial cells provide support and nutrition to the neurons. This could be the secret of the superb intelligence of Einstein.

The average weight of the human brain is 1300-1400 gm. The cerebellum contributes 142 gm. The brain consumes a lot of energy. It takes 20% of the total oxygen and glucose that the body consumes. This is the reason why the brain is richly supplied with blood about – 750-1000 ml/minute.

The nerve fibres are covered by a sheath called myelin sheath. The brain and spinal cord are two major parts of the central nervous system. The brain has three major divisions the forebrain the midbrain and the hindbrain.

The forebrain houses the thalamus and hypothalamus deeper in the neocortex and is responsible for motor control relaying the sensory information and also controlling autonomic functions (sympathetic and parasympathetic).

The midbrain and the hindbrain together are called the brainstem. The midbrain is involved in the functions of vision and hearing as well as motor functions.

The hindbrain is at the junction of the midbrain and beginning of the spinal cord. It is formed by the pons medulla oblongata and cerebellum.

Realizing the importance of the brain nature has made some special provisions for the brain. It is very nicely protected in a strong bony skull very hard to crack thus providing very solid protection from trauma. In addition to the bony protection the brain is also protected by three membranes and circulating fluid in between them. The outer most covering, the Dura is a very thick and tough membrane. A thin membrane, the arachnoid lines the dura from inside. The third thin layer is the pia mater. It rests directly on the surface of the brain and spinal cord is comparatively delicate and covers the cerebral cortex and carries the blood vessels to the brain. Cerebro spinal fluid between the arachnoid and pia mater forms a buffer and also provides some nourishment. This is one of the great wonders of nature.

No part of brain is less important than the other but there are a few areas of the brain which are of interest to an inquisitive common man. Let us discuss those smaller areas of more significance.

Broca's Area

The Broca's area is the name given after the scientist Paul Broca. It is commonly situated in the left (dominant) cerebral hemisphere in the inferior frontal gyrus. It is the speech and language center of the brain. It is also responsible for initiating complex patterns of bodily movements. In case it is attacked by a tumor the slow destruction of this area takes place but speech is still left relatively intact as the function of Broca's area is taken up by the neighboring area of the brain.

Carl-Wernicke's Area

This is situated at the junction of the temporal and parietal lobe. It is also linked to speech like the Broca's area. It is mainly involved in the understanding of the written and spoken language. It is located in the dominant cerebral hemisphere in the superior temporal gyrus. Destruction of the Wernickes area results in receptive fluent aphasia i. e. inability to speak. This area lies close to the auditory cortex. This area appears to be uniquely important for the comprehension of speech and sounds. If the Wernickes area is damaged there is a difficulty in understanding language. The speech is fluent but loses meaning.

The Limbic System

The limbic system formed the entire brain in animals on the lower level of the ladder of evolution. It consisted of the amygdala which generates fear and rage and the hippocompus doing the job of encoding and retrieving information stored in the memory. The thalamus directs and modulates activity in the cerebral cortex of animals on a higher stage of evolution. Even after the brain evolved more and more, these older parts of the brain were retained by nature. In fact they were given added responsibilities. The hypothalamus has many special duties as a regulatory authority.

Regulatory Authority - Hypothalamus

The Hypothalamus is a small part of the brain situated below the large cerebral hemispheres well protected from all sides. It is less than 5 gm. in weight, the size of a beetle nut and pink in color because of the richer blood supply compared to the rest of the brain. This is the primitive (100 million years old) brain of the animals on the lower step of the evolutionary ladder. It carries out a lot many important functions in the human brain. It is armed with a very highly developed sensing system and extensive direct and indirect connections within the brain and the nervous system.

The hypothalamus acts as a regulatory body for many important functions like equilibrium, hunger, thirst and temperature. It also controls anger and fear. The hypothalamus co-ordinates the many centers of the brain 24 hours a day. It also controls the pituitary gland and through it the complete metabolism of the body and the growth and secondary sex characters. Temperature regulation of the body is achieved by stimulating pituitary and sympathetic nervous systems which leads to dilatation of the blood vessels of the skin, opening the sweat glands, and bringing down the temperature of the body. At the same time hypothalamus sends signals to increase the rate of respiration further increasing the heat loss. These mechanisms are triggered by 1/10th of a degree change in body temperature. On the other hand if the body temperature is lowered, the hypothalamus sends signals to the adrenal glands and liver to release more glucose in the body to give fuel to the muscles. Shivering is ordered, which again helps in heat generation by contraction of the muscles. Sweat glands are shut down and blood supply to the skin is reduced to reduce heat loss. Creation of goose flesh is another way of causing contraction of the small muscles at the root of the hair (erector pilae) which results in heat being produced.

If there is infection by bacteria it changes the sensitivity of the sensors so that the temperature of the body is raised (fever), which controls the growth of the bacteria by subjecting them to adverse temperature. When the purpose of controlling the bacteria is served, sweating is ordered to bring down the temperature back to normal.

Managing the water balance of the body is another important function of the hypothalamus. If the water content of the body drops blood becomes more salty. Pituitary is ordered to release more anti-diuretic hormone (ADH). This makes the kidneys reabsorb more water resulting in reduced water loss in in the form

Broca's Area, Wernicke's Area

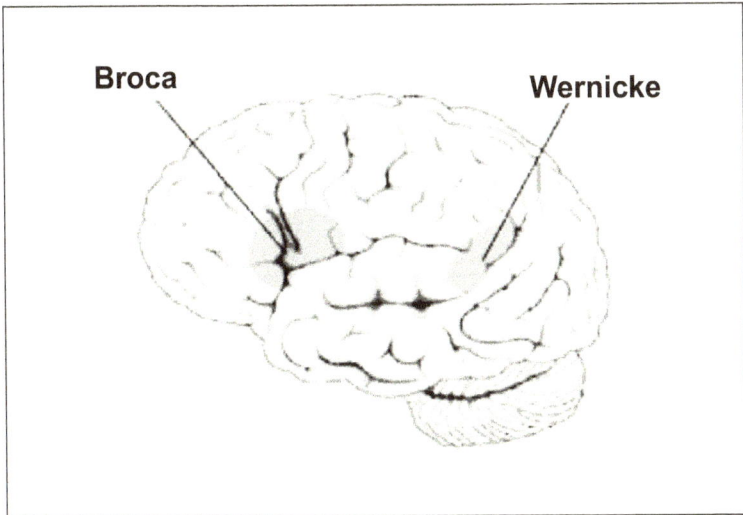

Broca   **Wernicke**

External Surface of Brain
Lobes Central Sulcus, Cerebellum, Spinal Cord

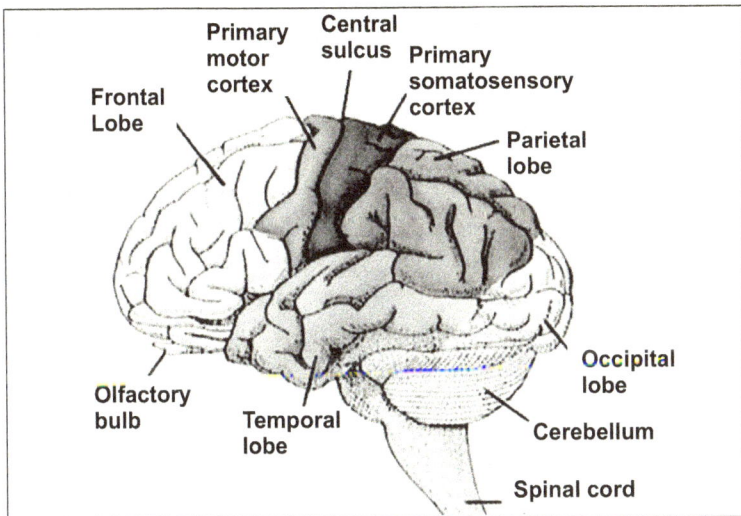

Primary motor cortex

Central sulcus

Primary somatosensory cortex

Frontal Lobe

Parietal lobe

Olfactory bulb

Occipital lobe

Temporal lobe

Cerebellum

Spinal cord

The Medial (Internal Surface)

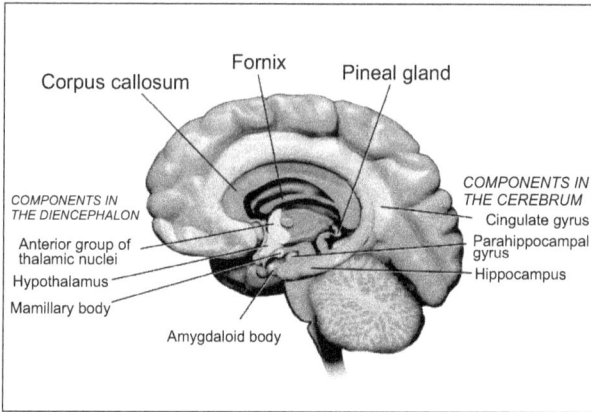

Corpus callosum
Fornix
Pineal gland

COMPONENTS IN
THE DIENCEPHALON
Anterior group of thalamic nuclei
Hypothalamus
Mamillary body
Amygdaloid body

COMPONENTS IN
THE CEREBRUM
Cingulate gyrus
Parahippocampal gyrus
Hippocampus

Limbic System

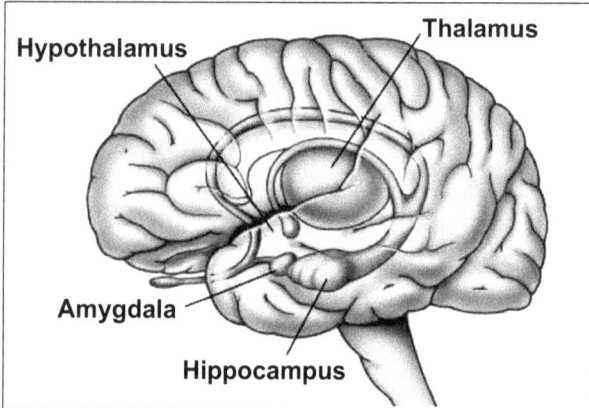

Hypothalamus
Thalamus
Amygdala
Hippocampus

Medial (Internal) Surface

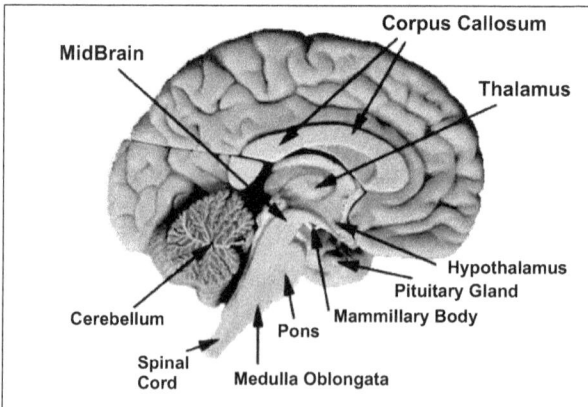

MidBrain
Corpus Callosum
Thalamus
Hypothalamus
Pituitary Gland
Mammillary Body
Cerebellum
Pons
Spinal Cord
Medulla Oblongata

of urine. The saliva secretion is also reduced which further contributes to the conservation of water. The hypothalamus creates thirst and sends an order to drink more water. On the other hand, increase in water content of blood signals pituitary to reduce ADH levels. This produces excessive loss of water in the form of urine.

Hunger

When blood sugar drops and fatigue is felt,the hypothalamus stimulates the contractions of the stomach, increases secretions of saliva and stomach, the taste buds become more sensitive, and we are given a message to eat. The person loses the satisfaction of eating if particular cells in the hypothalamus are damaged. He keeps on eating more. If the other type of cells are damaged we lose hunger sensation and interest in food.

Sex

The hypothalamus gives hormonal stimulation to the gonads (ovary or testicle). If certain cells are destroyed the sexual urge disappears. On the other hand irritation of these cells increases the desire for sex.

Temperament

Rage and fear act through the hypothalamus. It prepares us for a fight or flight response. This is done again through endocrine glands. The metabolic rate is increased, blood is directed from the skin to the muscles, breathing and heart beats are stepped up, and stomach activity is reduced; there is an urge to evacuate the bladder and bowel. Salivary glands are shut down leading to dryness of the mouth. If the rage or fear recedes, all these activities go in the reverse gear and the body comes back to normalcy.

This is one of the most important parts of the brain which is essential for survival.

I am tempted to give an analogy to the limbic system of King Bali an emperor depicted in an Indian mythological story. The story goes as follows.

King Bali was a very powerful king who was religious and altruistic as well. We all know that the human brain is adaptive and yet never satisfied with anything that is achieved. After winning the entire earth he thought of ruling the heavens. The gods in heaven were worried about a battle with him. Lord Vishnu came to the earth in the form of a poor short Brahmin boy 'Waman' by way of incarnation. He went to King Bali who was busy performing 'Yajnas' for conquering the heavens. Lord Vishnu in the form of the short Waman begged for space which could be covered by him within three steps. King Bali agreed to give it. Waman occupied the heaven in one step and the entire earth in the second. He asked King Bali where he should put his third step now. Bali bowed down and said meekly, "O Lord put it on my head." Waman put his third step on Bali's head and pushed him deep down under the earth to rule the land there.

The learned neocortex which came later has done exactly the same thing and pushed the limbic system deep down in the brain to rule at a lower level.

Auditory center

The auditory center is situated in the superior temporal gyrus of the brain. It perceives speech in association with the middle temporal gyrus.

Olfactory Center

Sensations are brought in by the olfactory bulbs, lateral olfactory tracts to the primary olfactory cortex then to the thalamus and on to the frontal cortex. This centre is the smell center.

Pons and Medulla

Pons and medulla are situated at the base of the cerebral hemispheres and is in front (anterior) of the cerebellum. Pons links the thalamus with the medulla. Nerve tracts linking the spinal cord and the cerebral cortex pass through the pons. Medulla is the lowest part of the brain stem which continues downwards as the spinal cord. The medulla does the most important role of regulating the heart beats, blood pressure and breathing.

Peripheral Nervous System

Brain the master needs many arms to serve it. The cranial nerves in twelve pairs, two from the fore brain and ten from the brain stem serve in receiving information from sensory organs such as the eyes, ears, nose, tongue and skin. Some of the cranial nerves have a motor function. They control the movements of the eye and the heart beats. In short, cranial nerves serve the head and neck.

The master is served by the somatic peripheral nerves for receiving touch, pain and temperature, vibrations from the skin muscles, bones and joints. These nerves come segmentally from the spinal cord. The motor nerves carry orders from the brain to all the muscles and glands.

Autonomic Nervous System

It is the one which controls predominantly functions which are largely not under voluntary control, such as heart beat, breathing, blood pressure, digestion and excretion, sexual arousal, salivation, perspiration pupillary reactions,and reflex actions like coughing, sneezing, swallowing and vomiting.

The autonomic nervous system is further divided in three parts - the sympathetic, parasympathetic, and the enteric nervous system.

One remarkable feature about the human body is the system of self-protection given to it by nature. It has provided protection to all the vital organs in order of the importance of their role for survival. The important abdominal organs are placed deep and protected by skin and muscles. Lungs and heart have been provided with a protective rib cage from the front and sides and by the vertebral column and strong muscles from the back. In the same way, the brain is protected with an almost invincible cranium made of very a thick and very hard bony covering from all the sides. The spinal cord is also protected by a very strong chain of vertebrae in its entire length. The brain is also covered by three membranes containing fluid in between them which provides good buffering action(acts as a good buffer).

Brain is not colorful. It is dull grey but it gets a sense of color with the help of the eyes. Beauty is said to be in the eyes of the beholder but not really so, it is a concept of the brain. Different brains see beauty in different things and persons.

This protection system is a blessing. Of course, it has its limitations and one day every being has to succumb to the all-powerful leveler, Death.

4 Third Eye

Pineal gland

The Pineal gland is a tiny gland from the endocrine system. It has the shape of a pinecone and the size of a wheat grain but has a much larger functional importance as compared to its size. It is situated between the two large cerebral hemispheres of the brain. The gland undergoes degenerative changes and becomes smaller in size as the child grows to the age of twelve years. Later in life it gets calcified because of the degenerative changes. Higher levels of fluoride in the blood hasten these changes. Tooth pastes containing fluoride, carbonated drinks, processed food, junk food, and use of non-stick pans for cooking raise the fluoride levels in the blood. The highest concentration of fluorides in the body is found in the pineal gland. Drinking purified filtered water and eating fresh organic food lowers the fluoride levels. Tamarind is also supposed to lower the fluoride levels. Sauna bath also reduces fluoride levels in the blood.

The pineal gland produces two hormones, the serotonin and melatonin. In fact, serotonin also acts as a precursor of melatonin. The hormone serotinin has a reproductive function. Higher levels of it can lead to the onset of puberty at an early age. Girls with this problem have a higher risk of getting breast cancer. The hormone melatonin is responsible for the circadian rhythm (sleep and wakefulness rhythm).

The eyes (retina) communicate a signal to pineal gland about light and darkness of the environment. In response the pineal gland keeps the levels of the hormone melatonin in the blood. Low levels of light in the bed room results in increased secretion of melatonin. This induces sleep. Higher or brighter light causes the opposite effect. This is what maintains the sleep and awakened state of man. That is why melatonin is used in medicine to treat depression and sleeplessness. Melatonin is very useful to prevent Jet lag. Tablet of melatonin is taken close to the target bed time of the destination. This gives satisfactory results.

Pineal gland is also termed the "Third Eye" because of its response to light like eyes. In mythological stories we read about the third eye of Lord Shiva. In western mythology also there are references to a third eye. I am a non-believer but believers link the pineal gland or the third eye to the metaphysical world. They think that this gland is the seat of the soul. A third hormone secreted by the pineal gland is Dimethyl tryptamine (DMT). This DMT is also called the "Spirit Molecule". Believers think that meditation rouses the third eye; it helps in meditation, emotional state of well being, time travel, journeys to paranormal realms and to encounters with spiritual beings from other dimensions. It is also thought to be the physical manifestation of the sixth Chakra of spiritual wisdom and thus the apparatus of spiritual vision which can take man between physical and metaphysical worlds. It allows him to have lucid dream experiences that are essential for spiritual evolution. In short, according to the believers, the pineal gland is the antenna designed to receive the messages from the spiritual world and the soul.

Pituitary Gland

Pituitary gland is the endocrine gland which is the master of the endocrine or hormone secreting glands. It is aptly called the master of endocrine orchestra, indicating that all the glands belonging to the endocrine system work in unison. The pituitary gland and most of the other endocrine glands have a biofeedback mechanism. They regulate the secretions of each other to maintain the required blood levels of the hormones secreted by the member glands of the orchestra.

The pituitary gland is about the size of a pea and weighs 0.5 gm in the human body. It is a protrusion off (protrudes from) the bottom of the hypothalamus at the base of the brain. It is well guarded in a bony-cavity called the pituitary fossa (sella turcica). It has three parts. The first is the posterior lobe that is functionally connected to the hypothalamus by a stalk called pituitary stalk. The anterior lobe is the second part which regulates several physiological processes by regulating the secretions of many endocrine glands (stress, growth, thyroid, reproduction, lactation etc.). The pituitary gland secretes nine hormones. The intermediate lobe is the third part which is only a few cell layers thick in humans. The endocrine cells of the anterior pituitary are connected to the hypothalamus by a portal system of capillaries which transport and exchange hormones to allow fast communication between both glands.

Hormones from the Anterior Pituitary

Growth hormone, prolactin, thyroid stimulating hormone, adrenocorticotropic hormone, melanocyte stimulating hormone, follicle stimulating hormone, and luteiningzing hormone are the hormones secreted by the anterior pituitary gland.

Tumors of pituitary gland are not very common, just 10% of all brain tumors. Majority of them are benign or non cancerous in nature. They can produce symptoms because of the pressure on the neighbouring optic nerve (nerve of the eye) and this leads to problems of vision or they produce different diseases because of reduced or increased secretion of a particular hormone. Hyper secretion of the growth hormone produces Gigantism and Acromegaly.

The pituitary diseases result from over-production or under-production of a particular hormone secreted by the pituitary gland. This usually results out of a benign tumor in some type of cells of the pituitary gland.

Anterior Pituitary Tumors

1) Acromegaly – Acromegaly results if there is an excessive production of growth hormone in adults. It is called gigantism in growing children. There is enlargement of hands, feet, lower jaw and brows. There may also be high blood pressure and diabetes.

2) TSH- Secreting Tumors – In this case the tumor cells produce excessive quantity of Thyroid stimulating hormone. It leads to symptoms of hyperthyroidism such as, weight loss in spite of increased appetite, palpitations, tremors, and anxious state of mind. These tumors are extremely rare.

3) ACTH- Secreting Tumors- Over production of ACTH produces mooning of the face (round face), weight gain and mental depression. This is known as Cushing's syndrome.

4) The tumors producing excessive follicular stimulating hormone, luteinizing hormone lead to infertility.

Posterior Pituitary Tumors

These are rare. They produce symptoms by pressing on optic

nerve and also cause a disease known as diabetes insipidus. The main symptoms are as follows - the patient passes large quantities of urine (low specific gravity – dilute urine) which leads to excessive loss of water from the body leading to excessive thirst.

Tests for Diagnosis

1) Blood levels of hormones

2) C.T. or MRI scans of the brain, with or without injecting a dye for contrast.

Treatments

Treatment of pituitary tumors needs a multi-disciplinary approach. The team consists of an endocrinologist, a neurosurgeon, a neuro-physician, an oncologist, and nurses trained in this field.

5 Master and Servants

Undoubtedly the brain is the master of the body. It controls everything in the body. Right from actions at cellular levels to gross interactions, emotions, thoughts, imagination, memory and experience - all are controlled by the master. Most of these actions appear to be voluntary. They are controlled by somato-sensory nerves. Digestion, excretion, blood pressure, heart beats, breathing and many other functions which seem to be involuntary, are also under the command of the brain through the autonomic nervous system.

Sensory nerves serve by bringing in sensations to the brain and are useful in learning about the internal and external environment. Motor nerves are the ones which carry the commands from the brain to the muscles and other organs and are responsible for the actions and responses of the body to the environment.

In case of the autonomic nervous system, both the sympathetic and the parasympathetic subtypes are under the control of the brain but not under volition. These functions are carried on automatically during sleep, unconsciousness, and even in coma. The nerves which bring in information are called afferent nerves and the ones which carry the command of the brain to the organs are called efferent nerves. The brain controls the important functions of digestion, excretion, maintaining blood pressure, heart beats and breathing. This goes on throughout life, round the clock, uninterrupted.

Neuropathy

The nerves from both the somato-sensory group and the autonomic group are prone to disease. They may be involved in isolation, in small or large groups. The process may be sudden (acute), or it may be gradual (chronic).

Thus, the damage or disease affecting nerves is called neuropathy. The effect may be on sensation, movement, glands or organ functions depending on the type of nerves affected. The common causes are diabetes, leprosy, vitamin deficiency, medication (chemotherapy),traumatic injury or excessive consumption of alcohol or tobacco. It can also be due to some inherited diseases, trauma, or because of immunological disease, or infections, viral as well as bacterial. It is also found in heavy metal poisoning. If a single nerve is involved, it is called mono-neuropathy, if many nerves are affected it is termed polyneuropathy.

Neuropathy may cause painful cramps, muscle twitching, muscle loss, bone degeneration, and changes in the skin hair and nails. Motor neuropathy may cause loss of balance and co-ordination. Sensory neuropathy may result in numbness to touch and vibration, reduced temperature sensation (Leprosy), reduced sense of position leading to poor co-ordination and balance. It can also cause spontaneous tingling or burning pain and pain from normally non-painful stimuli (light touch). Autonomic neuropathy leads to poor bladder control, abnormal blood pressure or heart rate.

Compression neuropathy is the result of abnormal pressure on a nerve e. g. carpal tunnel syndrome, axillary nerve palsy etc. The pins and needles sensation or the foot falling asleep is caused by temporary compression neuropathy. This can vanish with change of position and some movements. Direct injury to nerve or interruption of its blood supply or inflammation can also cause mono-neuropathy.

Poly-neuropathy is often serious as it affects more areas of the body. A common pattern (seen) in this is that the neurons are intact, but the axons (nerve fibers) are affected in proportion to their length. Diabetes is the most common cause of this type. The chief symptoms include weakness or clumsiness of movement (motor), unusual or unpleasant sensations such as tingling or burning, inability to feel texture and temperature. In sensory nerve involvement balance is impaired. When autonomic nerves are affected, the symptoms are dizziness on standing up, erectile dysfunction (sex), and difficulty in controlling urination.

Most of the neuropathies are slow in progress over months or years. In diabetes or pre-diabetic neuropathy such damage is often irreversible. Prevention is better than controlling the causative factor after the neuropathic changes have set in.

Some Common Causes

Endocrine disorders – diabetes, chronic renal failure, liver failure, heavy metals, excess of vitamin B-6, deficiency of vitamin B 1 and B 12 vitamin A and E. G. B. Syndrome, diphtheria, herpes simplex, herpes zoster, cancer radiotherapy, chemo all are among the causes of neuropathy.

Treatment

Antidepressants and antiepileptic drugs are found to be useful in managing neuropathic pain, e. g. Pregabalin, Amitriptyline,

Sodium Valproate, opiates and Digoxin.

Transcutaneous electrical nerve stimulation therapy may be useful in diabetic neuropathy.

Neutro Toxins (Survival of the Fittest)

Once we accept the concept of the food chain in nature, we know that all life forms are both prey and predators. The prey and predator relationship exists between plants, insects, the aquatic

> Diabetes should be prevented by exercise, controlling weight, and treating it at the earliest.

life forms and all the complex life forms on earth including the intelligent human race.

Plants are helpless in running away from predators but are not defenseless. They have their own way of protecting themselves by different means including producing toxic substances. Curare, a plant alkaloid paralyses the nervous system of animals and humans when it enters the blood. Men as hunters in jungles, and warriors of the bow and arrow era were aware of this neurotoxic property of curare and used it for application to the tip of their arrows. It is known to produce paralysis of all muscles, including muscles of respiration, thus killing the prey by asphyxia.

Some fishes (puffer fish), if not prepared correctly before eating, can invite death as it contains tetradotoxin (TTX). This tetradotoxin stops ions from flowing through the ion channel across the cell membrane by acting as a plug. Without the movement of sodium ions across the neuronal membrane, neurons are not able to send signals for communication to the nervous system properly.

It is only well known that snakes like the King Cobra and certain other reptiles and lizards also use a poison to paralyze and kill their prey or enemy. These are some of the ways used by predators to kill their prey by using neurotoxins.

Neurotoxins

Similarly exogenous compounds can prove toxic when they attain a critical concentration in the body. The examples are glutamate, nitric oxide, botulinum toxin, tetanus and tetradotoxin.

These neurotoxins inhibit neuron control over ion concentrations across the cell membrane or block communication between neurons across a synapse. They can cause glial cell damage. Neurotoxicity results in intellectual disability, memory impairments, epilepsy (excitotoxicity), and dementia. Antioxidants and antitoxins help reduce or reverse these damages.

Neurotoxins by definition are an extensive class of exogenous neurological chemicals which can adversely affect function in both developing and mature nervous tissues.

The nervous tissue has a very wide surface area for the neurons. They have a high lipid content which can retain liophilic toxin. Disproportionately rich blood flow to the brain increases the vulnerability of the nervous system to the neurotoxins. As the neurons last almost for the life time, the damage by toxins can be compounding. This brings us to nature's ways of providing protection to the brain. Blood can carry a host of ingested toxins. They must be prevented from reaching the brain. This is achieved by protective cells (astrocytes) around the capillaries in the brain. These astrocytes absorb the toxins from the blood and protect the brain cells from damage. This is known as Blood Brain Barrier (BBB). In addition to the BBB the choroid plexuses in the third, fourth and lateral ventricles secrete the cerebro-spinal fluid (CSF). These choroid plexuses allow the selective passage of ions and nutrients while trapping heavy metals like lead and mercury thus preventing damage to the brain cells.

Another class of neurotoxins causes hyper stimulation instead of paralysis. The hyper stimulation can cause tonic convulsions (as in tetanus), exhaustion, raised blood pressure and burst lung syndrome or pulmonary oedema.

The slowly acting neurotoxins can shorten the life of the neurons and contribute to neurodegenerative diseases like Alzheimers, Huntington's Chorea, and Parkinsonism.

Common Sources of Neurotoxins

Our food, water and air pollutants carry neurotoxins in concentrations which gradually damage the neurons. Junk food, baby food, artificial sweeteners used for diet or diabetes, aerated diet drinks (colas), chips, canned foods, chlorinated water, fluoride tooth pastes, antacids, vaccines contain aluminum. Fish products, Silver filling (dental), drinking water carry mercury in the body. Sodium caseinate in dairy products, junk food, yeast extract in processed food, canned food are all toxic to brain.

Precautions

Find pure food without pesticides, water without chlorine (Boiling is the best way to purify water).

Don'ts

Avoid fluoride tooth paste, choose foods without additives, and avoid all artificial sweeteners, vanilla, artificial colors in food products. Avoid processed and packaged food. Stay away from pesticide sprays. Minimize electromagnetic device uses.

Do's

Find pure food (difficult job). Drink plenty of water (filtered or boiled). Eat organic food as far as possible.

While thinking of all these do's and dont's it seems it is a difficult proposition to live in the present age without consuming these neurotoxins. We should at least strive to keep away from the dont's as far as possible.

6 Child's Play

The Baby's Brain

When we discuss an easy task to be performed, we call it child's play. We mean thereby that an adult can do it with little or no effort. However, in case of fast development of the brain and learning abilities the adults can be superseded by the embryo, foetus or a toddler. It is exclusively a child's play.

The development and growth of the fertilized ovum (the embryo) is fast. The brain and the entire nervous system develop from the embryonic layer called ectoderm. All the factors like wrong diet, consumption of tobacco, alcohol, infrared rays, X-rays, radiation, and cytotoxic drugs some chemicals including medicines taken by the mother during pregnancy can adversely affect the whole development of the foetus including the brain. The first ten weeks after gestation are very crucial from this point of view. The development of all the organs takes place fast but the last three months of intrauterine development and the first three years of life after birth show a phenomenal growth of the brain. It is estimated that the rate of growth of neurons (brain cells) is approximately 2.5 lakhs per minute. The electrical potentials of brain waves are detectable after forty days of gestation. The embryo after eight weeks is called the foetus; a miniature human form.

The pregnant woman should take good physical exercise, proper diet, enough sleep and have a good atmosphere around her. This is conducive to the good and healthy development of the foetus. The foetal brain starts learning a little but the real learning leading to experience and formation of memory starts after birth. It is understood that the development of the brain is seventy per cent completed before birth, about fifteen percent in the first year of life, and another ten percent up to the age of three years. The growth slows down at the age of twelve and almost stops after that age. It almost comes to a standstill after the age of 30 years.

It is also observed that the foetus can perceive smell and sound and can have perception of music to some extent. The foetus is capable of surviving with some help if delivered after six months. It is thought that the mind of the foetus can start functioning (existence) only after this stage.

Though the growth of neurons almost comes to a standstill after the initial year of life, the growth in the synaptic connections of the axons and dendrons continues till very late. The process of learning depends on both, the neurons of the brain and the synaptic connections. The neurotransmitters secreted at the synaptic connections are the actual mediators for transmission of impulses or messages from the periphery to the neurons and vice versa. The perception of pain, pleasure, smell, taste, vision, hearing, touch and any other sense organs has to go through these chemical mediators or the neurotransmitters. A rise or fall in the levels of this neurotransmitter can lead to impairment which may be responsible for the functional disorders or diseases of the brain and the nervous system.

The learning process starts on a smaller scale in intrauterine life.

The growth in the number of neurons and the innumerable synaptic connections which is remarkably rapid in first three years is instrumental in very fast learning of languages, skills and social awareness or creating the awareness of the surroundings as a whole. Reading for the child and later cultivating a reading habit in the child also

The new born learns earlier if the parents and siblings play and interact with the newborn. Ambience of music, healthy surroundings, emotional support, caring attendance, even respect for the newborn go a long way in the development of the child into a confident personality.

contribute immensely to the learning of the child. The child also learns from experiences in life.

Breast feeding by the mother gives the baby a sense of security and attachment to the mother and is the best food on the earth for the newborn. It also offers passive immunity which the baby has yet to develop. Breast feeding for at least a year is ideal.

Food supplements can be started three months after birth. The taste for different kinds of food starts developing by around the sixth month. This is the reason why the mother should start giving food supplements which would be healthy and be cultivated as a diet for the rest of life. Vegetable soups, fruit juices and rest of the food items should be started in small quantities, and in steps. Babies also have likes and dislikes for tastes. A mother should taste the food before giving it to the babies. Babies relish change in the taste of food, surroundings, background and even music. If these are conducive, they take the food quickly and get the satisfaction of eating.

Sound Mind In A Sound Body- Exercises

It is aptly said - 'sound mind in a sound body'. It is also true the other way round if the mind is sound the body also stays sound. A disturbed mind invites many diseases called psychosomatic disorders. Similarly a diseased body leads to fatigue, irritability, anxiety and depression. In short, the body and mind is a single unit. Naturally disturbance in one is bound to disturb the other.

Even our ancestors knew that physical exercise gives a healthy and sound body but as of late scientists have proved that physical exercise increases the blood supply to the brain and gives mental relaxation along with physical relaxation after exercise. Games in particular, help in focusing the mind. This helps to concentrate on tasks taken up by the brain like studies. Physical and mental relaxation through meditation is also conducive to good brain functioning. Physical and mental exercise both help in the development and growth of the brain and good functioning of the developed brain.

Antidepressant drugs like fluoxetine act by increasing the serotonin level. Regular exercise also boosts serotonin levels. Obviously physical exercise acts as a better antidepressant than drugs and should be preferred. Intense exercise helps secretion of endorphins which act as physiological mood elevators. These levels are sustained for a long time.

This explains the pleasurable, and even addictive nature of activities like running and swimming. Physical fitness increases the confidence for having sexual activity and also the pleasure one gets from it. Exercises, along with an increase in the energy levels help to increase the self-esteem of the person.

This helps to improve memory, learning abilities, concentration and reasoning. Walking for 20 -30 minutes every day preferably

The cognitive abilities of the neocortex are also seen to increase with physical exercises like walking. This is attributed to the increased supply of oxygen and glucose to the brain.

at the designated time is useful. This has been proved by controlled trials on groups. The least that can be easily done is to flex and extend the toes of the feet and the ankles while going to bed, walking in the morning or even after an hour's sitting.

In Alzheimer's disease, the neurons die for want of use. Exercise helps to keep alive the neurons in the hippocampus which delay the symptoms of Alzheimers. Earning new physical as well as mental skills through puzzles, chess, bridge and outdoor games help by increasing blood supply as well as by stimulating memory skills. Going for treks and outings to scenic places exposes us to a variety of experiences and makes us think about them. This is also a very rich brain stimulant.

Dr. Lorence Cart (Dukes University) has suggested an exercise called neurobics. It gives an integrated stimulus to physical and emotional faculties. You are taught to do some of the routine tasks with eyes closed and use sign language instead of talking. You are trained to use multiple tasks simultaneously using different sense organs. Cleveland clinic has shown that physical strength of your muscles can be increased by imagining that you are doing a physical exercise. This also helps in improving the function of the neo- cortex to some extent.

Physical activity done during the course of routine work is not exercise. It is the physical activity done deliberately in leisure time. At the same time the person doing exercise must pay attention or apply the mind to the exercise. Regularity in the exercise pays. Strenuous exercise done erratically is counterproductive. Static exercises like weight lifting dumbbells pressing or stretching springs are also useful. Surya Namaskar an Indian exercise belongs to this category. It builds up muscle strength and gives good shape to the body. 12-15 minutes of this exercise thrice a week is recommended.

Kinesthetic Exercises

Along with muscle movements, movements of joints through walking, running, playing games, cycling and swimming fall in this category. This should be done for about 30 minutes 3-5 days a week. This exercise increases the efficiency of the heart lungs and prevents obesity. It keeps blood sugar in control, drives away depression improves digestion and gives sound sleep.

Yoga

Yoga helps more for keeping the elasticity of muscles and ligaments and helps keep the balance of the body. Surya Namaskar and P.T. exercises in schools also fall under this category. It is recommended for 10-15 minutes thrice a week.

Endurance Building

In this category of exercise we aim at building endurance without physical fatigue. Doing brisk walking or cycling for 40 minutes daily is always good.

Regularity is the essence of exercise. A little background music avoids the feeling of monotony. Medical advice about choice and duration of exercise should be sought especially by the elderly and those suffering from some illness or pain.

"Junk Food Junks the Brain" - DIET

The food to be given to a pregnant woman has been a hot topic of discussion in medical literature. In fact a lot of attention and care always went into the selection of food for pregnant women in the ancient times. We are giving an explanation for selecting these food items in the light of the modern research. Knowledge of micro-nutrients such as vitamins, minerals, calories per gram of proteins, carbohydrates and fats may be of recent origins. The understanding of the utility of fibers in the diet has been acquired recently but the age-old methods of selection of food were well thought of.

The fancy for the fast food the junk food, is of a comparatively recent origin. All the diet experts are shouting for quite some time and condemning the use of junk foods but to no avail. It has been proved beyond doubt that junk food leads to obesity. The atherosclerosis and the attendant risk factors of high blood pressure diabetes mellitus both of which contribute to diseases of the heart, liver, brain, kidneys and cancers are pointed out by experts. All of these devils are increasing the morbidity and mortality of human beings. Junk foods are converting human bodies into junk yards. Junk food taken by mothers in pregnancy is harmful for the health of the babies in the womb.

The route taken by the junk food for destruction of health is through the genes and through the brain. The younger generations are almost getting addicted to junk food before gaining knowledge about their hostility. The regulating authorities have started a system to warn the people about consumption of tobacco by using health hazard warnings. Time has come to give such warning for junk food and may be bringing up ordinances to curb or stop the use of harmful diets.

With these opening remarks let us go to the discussion of what should be the contents of an ideal diet.

The genetic messages and the development of the organ system and the brain largely depend on what the embryo gets from the father in genes and from the mother in genes and nourishment. This brings us to the discussion of the all important diet of the mother. If this diet is deficient or defective it is in all probability going to create problems to the baby to be born before and after birth.

It was thought that the genes cannot be changed but proper nourishment could be provided to the foetus. In fact now with a lot of research in the genes the epigenetics and the methods of genetic engineering, scientists are giving hope to mankind that it would be possible to change the defective genes or prevent them from expressing in the next generation so that things like diabetes, heart diseases and cancers may be prevented in gen next in the near foreseeable future.

I am restricting the discussion on diet to nurturing of the brain and the nervous system in particular with passing remarks for health in general.

Diet of the Mother

If we pay attention to the diet of the mother after detecting pregnancy it may be a late awakening. If the same attention is given to the prospective mothers it has a lot of advantages. Take a simple example. If the prospective mother has deficiency of the vitamin folic acid and if she realizes that she is pregnant (4-6 weeks) the embryo is likely to develop some neural tube defect. The neural tube goes to form the brain and the nervous system. Babies with neural tube defect are likely to have menigocele or menigomyelocele with defects in both the lower limbs and control of bowel and bladder almost permanently. Pediatricians and neo-natologists are recommending that all the prospective mothers should be given a tablet of folic acid every day before they plan pregnancy.

The important factors for the healthy development of the brain and the nervous system of the foetus are Omega 3 fatty acids Docosahexaenoic Acid (DHA), arachidonic acid, BComplex vitamins, Folic acid, Vitamin-C, Vitamin-E, iodine, iron, zinc celenium, amino acids – choline and antioxidants from raw salads cucumber carrots tomatoes and onions.

The mother should start taking these prospectively when pregnancy is being planned should continue it in pregnancy and lactation. Balanced diet containing requisite amount of proteins carbohydrates and fatty acids should be included in the mother's diet during pregnancy and lactation. Milk must be taken in adequate quantity. Taxin is very useful for the development of retina of the eye. It can be sourced through meat eggs and fish. Vegetarians can use plenty of milk. Folic acid and vitamins can be sourced through leafy vegetables, pulses, liver, yeast and citrus fruits, zinc from cherry, mango, pomegranate, tomatoes, onion leaves, carrot, beet and potatoes. Iron from green leafy vegetables eggs, meat, *chiku*, pineapple, *Haliv*, sesame, *karale*, dates, almonds, pistachio, almonds and sprouted pulses. Iodine can be sourced from fish, pulses and iodized salt. *Haliv laddoos* with all dry fruits given to pregnant women in Indian culture cover most of the requirements.

In short, a brain-friendly diet must be given to the pregnant ladies and a growing infant. If selected carefully from the available food stuffs it is not costly. In case this food does not contain one of the items recommended, a supplement in the form of a multivitamin mineral pill is handy.

7 Brain Image

Every human being tries to project a good image of himself or herself. So far as the master controller, the brain is concerned, it is shy of projecting its own image unless lured by light or magnetic energy. However doctors need to have brain images when there is some problem with or disorder in the brain. The following are some ways to check the problem so that it can be solved and the person can be healthy. His health depends heavily on the brain.

The age old X-ray imaging invented by Roentgen in 1895 gives very little information of the brain. The Computed Tomography (C.T) a new form of X-ray imaging developed by Godfrey Hounsfield (1972) gives an integrated and reconstructed image of the brain analysed by the computer. The introduction of CT proved very useful in neurological diagnosis. The diagnosis of blood clots, brain tumors has been easy with CT. Digital Subtraction Angiography (DSA) is a method in which a radio-opaque dye (contrast) is injected into a blood vessel. Once this contrast reaches the brain, X-rays are taken. The image is obtained by subtracting the unwanted image of bones and soft tissues so that doctors can get a clear view of the blood vessels filled with the contrast. This gives a beautiful picture of the vascular (arterial) tree of the entire brain at a time. It becomes easy to find out Artrio-venous malformations (AVM), aneurysms and abnormal vascular patterns of the brain tumors or abscess.

PET Scan

Positron Emission Tomography involves emission of positrons from an isotope in a tracer dose given through injection or inhalation. The positrons are neutralized by electrons in the body tissue that release energy in the form of radiation. This radiation produces the image. This is useful to see the blood flow or the metabolic activity in different areas of the body. This can give us clues about the abnormalities in the body. This is a costly procedure.

Spect

Single Photon Emission Computed Tomography is a less expensive method than PET Scan for obtaining two and three-dimensioned reconstruction of brain blood flow.

MRI

MRI is Magnetic Resonance Imaging. Harshad Godbole has written an informative article on MRI in Lokmat dated 20.8.2014. Raymond Damadian postulated the theory that magnetic waves can be used for diagnosis of diseases like cancers or abnormalities. In 1977 he constructed a machine for body scanning for cancer. It was called Nuclear Magnetic Resonance (NMR) machine. Now it is known as MRI (Magnetic Resonance Machine)

The patient is placed within a magnetic coil and then radio frequency energy is applied to the body. The harmless radio waves are useful for imaging without radiation. MRI is an excellent modality to evaluate the soft tissues of the body, the brain and the spine.

Role of Interventional Radiology, (IVR) is used in case of brain stroke for thrombosis of an artery supplying part of the brain. Strokes caused by blood clots can be treated by intra-arterial thrombolysis within six hours from the start of the symptoms. Intra-arterial thrombolysis is carried out by threading a fine tube (micro catheter) from the groin to the blocked artery in the brain and then injecting clot dissolving substances. Similarly a clot in the vein of the brain can be treated.

Brain Image PET.CT & PET MRI

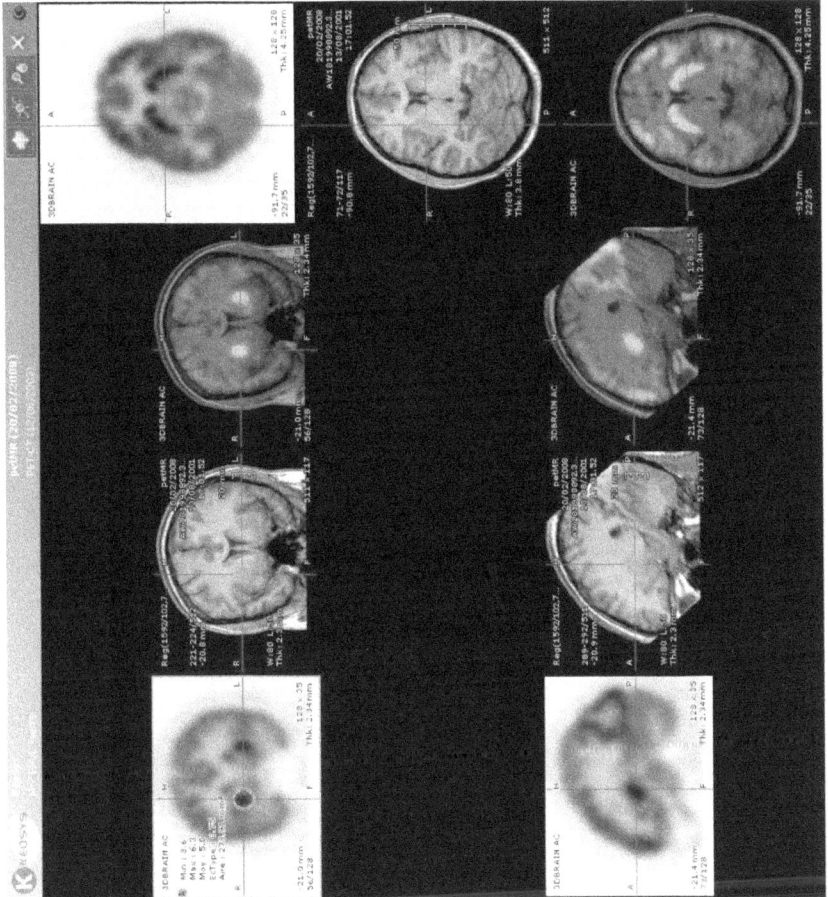

DSA Brain

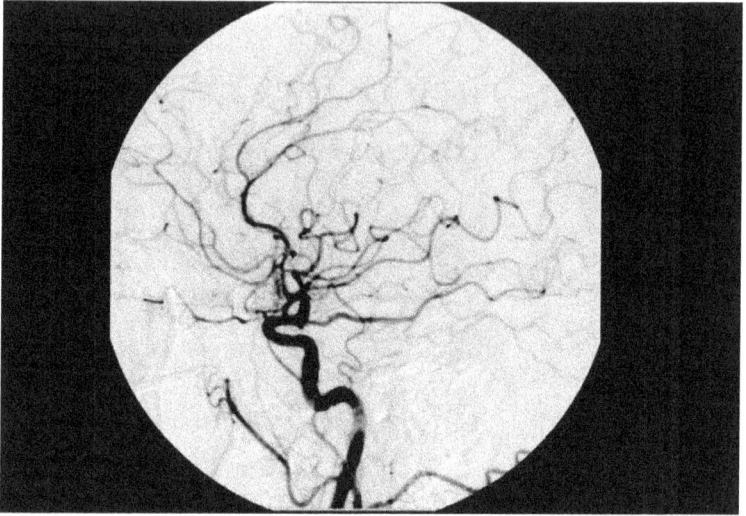

MRI

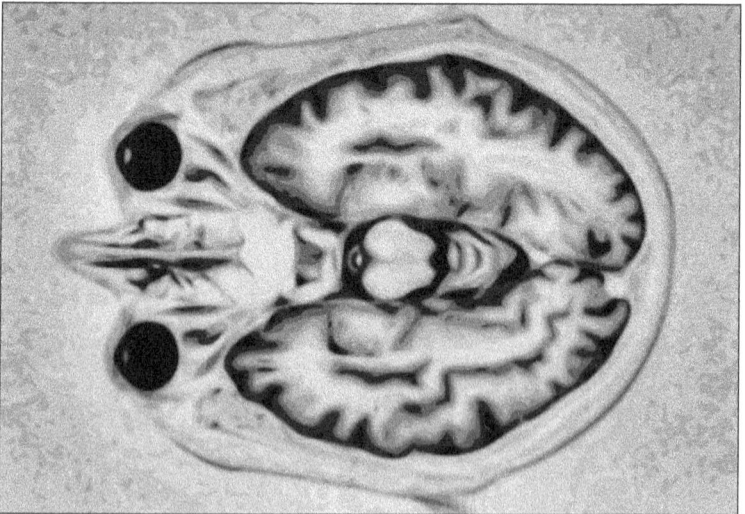

Spina Bifida Meningocoele

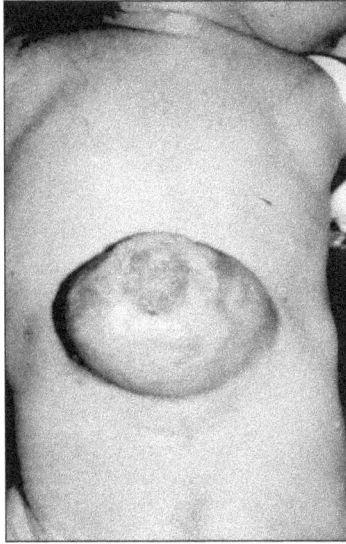

Encephalocoele

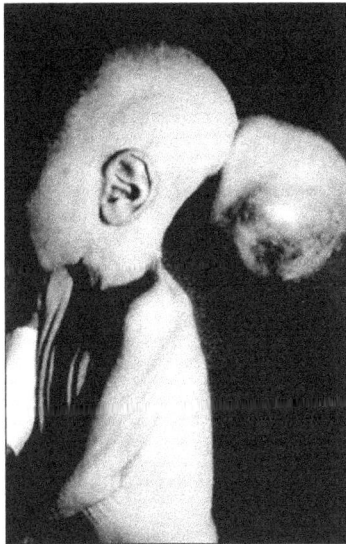

Note : This is easily avoidable by taking precautionary measures

Anencephaly

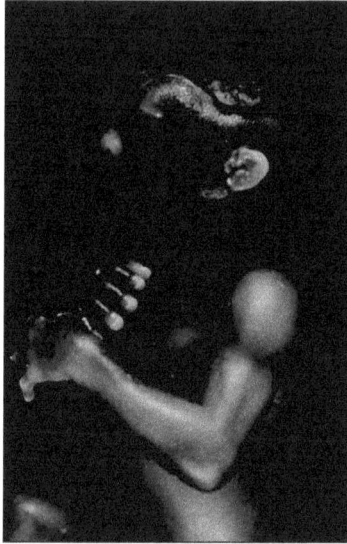

Alien Head (Hydrocephalus)

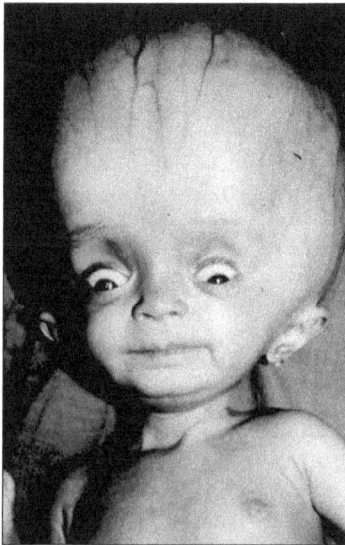

Note : This is easily avoidable by taking precautionary measures

8 Prince Without A Crown Seat

Anencephaly

Brain is the crowned king of the human body. Sometimes the prince is born but may lack the seat of the crown. The brain may not have developed at all hence the Cranial vault is also missing. It is understandable when there is no valuable item, the safe deposit vault is not necessary. When the brain is completely missing at birth it is called Holoanencephaly. At times the brain is substituted by abnormal spongy vascular tissue admixed with glial cells (no neurons) the condition is called Meroanencephaly. Both of these do not survive.

Anencephaly is more common than, Holo and Meroanencephaly is the where a major portion of the brain skull and scalp are absent at birth. It is the result of the neural-tube defect at the head end. The largest part of the brain mainly the cerebral hemispheres including the Neo-cortex which distinguishes human beings from rest of the animal world is missing. is the requirement of cognition.

The remaining brain is often exposed for want of cranial vault and the scalp. Most of such babies do not survive. Those with these covers intact are likely to survive for some time with learning disabilities and without many humanly faculties. They may be blind deaf and unaware of their surroundings. Because the brainstem is intact, breathing and responses to sounds or touch may be present.

The highest point of the skull of such babies is occupied by the eyes giving them a look of frog head. They have no brain the crown of intelligence and the cap.

There is no concrete proof about any genetic defect responsible for this defect. Mothers taking anti-epileptic drugs or insulin for diabetes are more prone to give birth to such children. Addition of Folic acid 4 mg a day to the diet of the mother has been seen to prevent many defects of the neural tube in babies if it is given prospectively. If the mother is exposed to high levels of toxins such as lead, chromium, mercury and nickel this also predisposes to anencephaly.

Microcephaly

This is the under development of the brain. It is usually defined as head circumference 2-3 standard deviations below the mean for age and sex.

Microcephaly may be present at birth or it may develop in the first few years of life. It may be due to chromosomal abnormality or due to disruptive injuries, ischemic stroke, haemorrhagic stroke or congenital infections or maternal exposure to radiation – during pregnancy or poorly controlled diabetes of the mother and placental insufficiency. There may be many more diseases which can damage the foetal brain in its developmental stage.

Affected newborns have major neurological defects, seizures and severely impaired intellect. Motor functions of muscles may appear later. The head size at birth may be normal or small but soon the head fails to grow while the face continues to grow-normally. As the child grows the head appears proportionately smaller. There is no specific treatment.

Birth Defects of the Brain and Nervous System

There are some preventable congenital defects of brain. The defect in the head end of the neural tube leads to failure of development of the parts of the brain especially the neo-cortex acquired lately in the process of evolution. They include anencephaly microcephaly and menigocoeles of head and neck. Hydrocephalus is another developmental defect at the head

Brain and the nervous system develops from the ectoderm which is the embryonic layer from which the skin of the embryo also develops. An infolding and formation of a tube from the ectoderm which goes to form the neural tube is the precursor of the entire nervous system. Any defect in the neural tube leads to congenital anomalies of the brain or spinal cord.

end. A defect in the caudal or lower end of the neural tube results in the formation of menigocle myelomenigocoele and spina bifida at the lumbosacral end of the spine (back).

Alien Head - Hydrocephalus

In many science fiction stories and films we see a typical picture of an alien. The head is very large in proportion to the entire body and face. There is no hair on the scalp of aliens. The eyes, nose, ears mouth and chin all are very small as compared to the head.

This is the exact picture of obstructive hydrocephalus when it occurs in a baby before the fontanelle and the suture joint of the skull bones unite that is before the age of 2-3 years.

Hydrocephalus is a medical condition of excessive accumulation of cerebrospinal fluid (C.S.F.) in the cavities (ventricles) of the brain. This causes increased intracranial pressure leading to the enlargement of the head.

If untreated this leads to mental disability, tunnel vision and convulsions leading to death. Let us try to understand the reasons leading to this problem.

C. S. F. is the fluid secreted by the specialized cells in the brain. This fluid circulates through all the cavities (ventricles) of the brain and bathes the brain and the spinal cord. It provides part of the nourishment to the nervous tissues and takes some of the unwanted products of metabolism and toxins away from the nervous tissue. In addition it gives a very sound buffering protection to the brain from trauma. This C.S.F. is having a place of production path of circulation with some bottle necks on the way and is ultimately reabsorbed by the arachnoid villi into a venous channel.

Excessive production, obstruction in the path of circulation or difficulty in re-absorption can lead to increase in the amount of C.S.F. in the system leading to rise in intra cranial pressure. This high pressure leads to increase in size of the head. If this problem occurs before the fontanelle and the suture joints of the skull bones have united after birth (2-3 years of age) the skull (head) increases in the size out of proportion. The rest of the body including the entire face also is growing at normal pace or in fact at a retarded rate because of the problem to the brain. This gives the baby a look of the typical alien figure depicted in science fiction films.

The most common cause is the obstruction to the flow of the C.S.F. in the aqueduct of sylvius or in the inter-ventricular (foramina) communications. Another type is non obstructive. Here there is an abnormal increase in production of C.S.F. or defective (reduced) reabsorption of C.S.F. by the arachnoid granulations located along the (superior saggital sinus) a venous sinus.

Besides the congenital causes the obstruction to the flow of C.S.F. may be caused by viral, bacteria, tubercular infections in the newborn sometimes it can be due to a tumor.

The head enlarges in size only if the hydrocephalus develops before the age of 3 years i. e. before the skull bones are united.

Clinical Picture

The infant exhibits fretfulness, poor feeding, frequent vomiting and lack of interest in his surroundings later. The upper eyelids become retracted and eye balls turn down. ("Sunset eyes")

Acquired Hydrocephalus

When infections, brain tumors, head trauma and intracranial bleeding cause obstruction and if the skull bones are already fused it is very painful because of the high intracranial pressure, severe headache, vomiting and neurological deficits show in.

Treatment

The treatment of hydrocephalus is only surgical. Where ever there is an obstruction bye-pass is the treatment. A small caliber silastic tube (catheter) is put into the ventricle of the brain and the other end is put into another body cavity from where the C.S.F. can be reabsorbed. The commonest shunt is with the peritoneal cavity (abdomen), pleura (around lung), lt atrium of the heart or gall bladder.

Complication

After surgery if there is infection or blocking of the shunt it may warrant a repeat surgery.

Spina Bifida

The incomplete closure of the embryonic neural tube also causes failure of the closure of the spines of the vertebrae hence it is called spina bifida. As the spine is not closed at the back the meniges and/or the defective spinal cord may bulge through the defect. It often forms a cystic sac called meningocole or myelomeningocoele. When the defect is mild it is covered with skin. There may or may not be a neurological defect. If the defect is large and results in menigocoele or myelomeningocoele there may be mild to severe neurological problems below the waist. There may be a defective bladder and bowel control. In addition there can be defects in the lower limbs such as club foot hip dislocation and scoliosis.

Surgery done during foetal life or in the neonatal life can be of use to a varying degree depending upon the severity of the problem and the neurological defects already present.

Prevention

A large number (73%) of these congenital defects of the brain and the nervous system are preventable. The neural tube defects such as Anencephaly Hydrocephalus and spina bifidas can be prevented by giving a tablet of folic acid daily to the prospective mother. Once the couple makes a decision to have a baby the lady should start a tablet of folic acid daily 3 months prior to stopping the family planning measures. If the lady starts folic acid after she realizes that she is pregnant it is too late to prevent these defects. The cost of the 5 mg tablet of folic acid is 25 paise which is well within the reach of a common man.

Anaemia in the mother can also lead to slowing down the progress of the mental faculties of the brain. Prevention or correction of anaemia in the prospective mother and delaying the clamping of the umbilical cord for 2 minutes before cutting can go a long way in preventing this problem. Green and leafy vegetables are a rich source of iron and folic acid. It can help in preventing both types of problems.

9 TheMind – An Enigma

What do we exactly mean by mind? Can you see the mind? Can you locate a particular area in the brain or in the body where the mind dwells? The answers to these questions are not easy. The 'Gita' says that mind is the sixth organ but this mind is not visible. We cannot pinpoint a centre in the brain where it stays but we can infer that mind is a faculty of a living brain. Probably memory thinking, experience and many other things have to come together to make the mind. The sum of many faculties leads to the concept of the mind. You cannot peep into the mind of others. It is a very closely guarded secret. Neuroscientists are working hard to peep in the mind but have met with very little success as yet. The only reasonable way of understanding somebody's mind is to watch the person's actions, expressions and body language and hear his speech. We have to study the overall behavior of the person and guess what the person has in his mind. Leave aside another person do we understand our own mind fully and all the time? Probably not. Sigmund Freud says that the mind is like an iceberg it floats with one-seventh of its bulk above water. The mind or the faculties of the mind such as thinking and imagination have no boundaries. It is not confined to the skull or the body. It can be here, now and it may be on the Moon or Mars or anywhere in the universe in less than a fraction of a second. It is limited only by our knowledge and imagination.

I agree with Maulana Wahiduddin Khan when he says "Mind is the Architect of Personality" [Times of India - Speaking tree 13.9.2014] "Not facility, not ease, but difficulty and efforts make a man or a woman," wrote the Scottish author and reformer Samuel Smiles.

All those greats, irrespective of their fields are made by the difficulties that came their way. They faced challenges and emerged as super achievers. The reason is traceable to one of the laws of nature. All our actions big or small are directly related to our minds. It is the mind that is the master of our personality as it controls all of our thoughts and activities. The mind has unlimited reserves of energy. If we have an easy job the mind releases lesser energy and if the task is difficult it releases greater amount of energy. If we are facing difficulties and are ambitious, the mind will make all out efforts to achieve the objective by releasing a greater energy, the result is we will develop a strong personality and will be achievers. This is the reason why we say that man is the master of his destiny. Thus every individual is self made. The quantum of success depends on this energy of the mind and proper planning of the efforts. We can be the mentor of the superman in us.

The mind seems to be very busy. Another question, in what stage of human life does the mind start working? Is it from the conception; is it in foetal life or at some time after birth? Certainly not from conception as the brain is not formed till a few weeks after conception. The mind of the foetus starts working on a limited scale at a later stage of foetal life probably after a certain stage of development of the brain. The movements like sucking of

The learning process starts on a fast track only after the birth. The first few years after birth are really fast. The function of the mind blossoms with increasing knowledge of the world around. Then it cruises at a speed much faster than any physical mode of travelling at our disposal today.

the thumb or playing with the roommate (twin), responding to music may be thought of as a limited activity of the brain and mind as well.

This is the speed of imagination of the mind. The mind works relentlessly till death possibly barring exceptions of deep coma or unconscious state. This brings us to a discussion on what is consciousness and what is unconsciousness.

Consciousness

What is consciousness? It is defined as a state of being conscious. The concept of Consciousness of the spiritualists is different than that of scientists. The men of science call it as a state of mind expressed by various faculties of thinking, speech taking logical decisions on the basis of learning and experiences and acting upon them. This is the consciousness of the biological life forms of all sorts. I believe despite the lack of a well defined nervous system or brain that the minutest unicellular life forms also possess consciousness essential for their survival and propagation. They have the basic intelligence limited for that purpose. That is the reason why they respond to unfriendly environment and go into hibernation and stay in their shell till the environment becomes friendly once again for restoring active life process and start propagating. If the environment is marginally hostile they respond by mutation instead of going into hibernation. Multi-cellular plants and animals also have intelligence and consciousness suited for their survival and propagation. Human beings are blessed with many facets of consciousness commensurate with their highly evolved status.

Animals have limited consciousness in that they also have the ability to perceive sensations and think of their survival and propagation.

They have intelligence required for getting food and water. They possess a sense of protecting their lives and propagating their D.N.A. They also exhibit some emotions in the limited sense. They show love and affection for their offspring and feed them till they become self-sufficient. However the faculties of speech, intelligence, memory, emotions and consciousness gifted to human beings are unique and phenomenal. It gives them a clear sense of identity. The dictionary meaning of consciousness is the state of being conscious.

It is very difficult to give a precise definition of consciousness. Consciousness is the product of many faculties of the brain working together in tandem giving us the knowledge of our own existence, sensations, cognitions, thoughts, feelings and emotions. Anything that we are aware of at any given moment is part of our consciousness. This may be for inner body activities or our surroundings. Even though consciousness springs from the brain the imaging techniques cannot pinpoint a seat of consciousness in a particular part of the brain. Computers are making big strides by imitating the neural network of the brain and doing many intelligent functions which were the sole prerogative of the brain. Scientists are optimistic. They believe that one day machines will be intelligent and perhaps conscious. Only time will tell. Nothing is impossible so let us keep our fingers crossed.

A living brain is required to be conscious. The brain has a physical form following the laws of physics chemistry and biology but consciousness and the mind do not follow any of these laws. When we see our favorite chocolate just the sight makes us happy because of our previous experience of its taste. We get a pleasant feeling in anticipation of the taste of the chocolate.

Philosophers of the world have expressed innumerable views on consciousness. Spiritualists define consciousness in a different way. They say that gaining consciousness is the acquisition of spiritual knowledge and state. Functionalists say that the brain is conscious because it is processing information in a particular way and consciousness is wholly non-material. Idealists on the other hand have a view that the mind or spirit is the only thing that exists. The material universe is the illusion produced by it. Shri Shankaracharya says that the world we call real is actually Maya or illusion and the reality is Brahma. Today neuroscientists are trying to discover how the activity of the brain cells translates into multifaceted experience of consciousness such as thoughts, perceptions, awareness and emotions. It is observed that consciousness occurs when certain brain cells fire in synchrony but strangely consciousness is lost if all the brain cells synchronise at the same moment.

Consciousness is assessed in the medical field by observing a patient's rising and responsiveness. If the patients have disorientation, delirium and loss of meaningful communication we say that their consciousness is impaired. Loss of movement in response to painful stimuli is termed loss of consciousness

So far as humans are concerned consciousness can be altered by trauma, illness, metabolic disorders and drugs. The states of sleep and coma alter consciousness. Consciousness can be easily restored from the state of sleep from the drug (Sedatives LSD etc) induced state with some efforts. It can be recovered with great difficulty from coma but consciousness ends after death never to return.

Unconsciousness

To put it in simple words it means a state of being not conscious. It characterizes a mental state where there is complete or near complete lack of responsiveness to people and to other environmental stimuli. There is a temporary loss of consciousness when man faints because of lack of supply of oxygen to the brain or when blood pressure falls or if there is asphyxia. In certain illnesses, the patient is delirious (only partially responsive to the surroundings). Persons in a state of sleep or hypnosis can however respond to stimuli fairly quickly.

> Today the internet has developed on an amazing scale. Will further development make it function consciously? Francis Heylighen argues that web pages are like information containing brain cells and the hyperlinks between them are like synaptic connections between brain cells.

The term unconscious is used not only for the fainting stage but also for thoughts deeper down which are not easily accessible. Our unconscious mind or subconscious is supposed to be unknown to our conscious. Researchers have concluded that a lot of unconscious processing goes a long way in the decisions of our conscious thinking and behavior. This may be compared to the overt action of a very sophisticated jet engine which needs a lot of coordinated pre-processing of innumerable individual small parts in order to produce the overt final action. In the engine there are multiple physical parts while in the unconscious processing they are innumerable functional elements working in harmony.

Sigmund Freud was one of the pioneers in psychology who put forth the importance of the unconscious mind. He related many of the psychological disorders to the suppressed sexual desires in the unconscious from infancy. This view is not accepted in the present day practice of psychiatry. However we are convinced about the important role of the unconscious mind in providing vital inputs to the conscious mind. Thus, our lives are ruled by thoughts and feelings of which we are not aware in a conscious state. Psychoanalysis is the technique used by the psychiatrists to dig out thoughts suppressed at unconscious level for cures. Preconscious or subliminal terms are used for experiences just below conscious thoughts.

Subconscious

In psychology the subconscious is the part of consciousness that is not currently in focal awareness. A psychologist Pierre Janet says, "Underneath the layers of critical thought functions of the conscious mind lie a powerful awareness that is the subconscious mind." He thinks that there is a limit to the information that can be held in conscious focal awareness. In short the subconscious is in the form of a store house of ones knowledge and prior experience. The terms subconscious and unconscious should not be used interchangeably. The term unconscious is far different from subconscious as used in the medical field.

Global Brain

If they arc thrown in search engines and other intelligent programs could it come alive? This is the idea of the Global Brain. It seems less probable if not impossible based on todays knowledge. The dream of a conscious and thinking machine is still a distant reality.

Some readers may have seen the article "Mind over Matter: Scientists find a way to email brainwaves" in SCI-Tech, Pune Mirror 30.8.2014 from the Times of India. A scientist in Thiruananthpuram transmits a message into the mind of a colleague 5000 miles away in France Strasbourg using brainwaves. Brainwave sensing machines have been used to telepathically allowing someone in India to send an e-mail to his colleague in France using nothing but the power of his mind. The researchers used electro-encephalography (EEG) headsets to record electrical activity from neurons firing in the brain and convert the words into binary reports. In EEG electrical currents in the brain are linked with different thoughts that are then fed into a computer interface. This computer analyses the signals and controls an action. In the latest study published in PLOS One researchers decided to replace the computer interface with another brain to receive the signals. A computer translated the message and then used electrical stimulation to implant it in the receivers mind. Participants did not report feeling anything in the process and only saw flickers of light in their peripheral vision.

The light appeared in sequences that allowed the receiver to decode the information in the message.

In such experiments there was an error ranging from 5 to 15%. Still this is a budding area of study. The Scientists say that in the near future computers will communicate directly with human brain in a fluent manner supporting both computer and brain-to-brain communication routinely.

Virtual Reality of The Mind

All our experiences, sights, sounds, smells, tastes and touch are in fact the interpretations of our mind about the realities around us. Without a mind to perceive it, a sound is a mere pattern of vibrations in the air. Thus, the perceptions of our mind are in essence an elaborate form of Virtual Reality

The light we see or the sound we hear are only a small part of the spectrum of light or sound that our senses can perceive and brain can interpret. It is interesting to note that our skin can be trained to send pulses of electricity that represent the shape of an object; the brain learns to interpret these signals as vision. Blind people are able to navigate their way with this technique. In short our skin can see.

Virtual reality is a great phenomenon about the brain. We need to be awake to experience consciousness. There are different states of consciousness. The dividing line between these states of consciousness and that leading to unconsciousness are thin and often blurred. The Human mind is capable of "Virtual Reality" from within like in dreams. Even in normal consciousness or in the absence of direct perceptions of the surroundings our thoughts and sensations can be the product of the brain. This power is the source of illusions and hallucinations.

The God Spot

One of the most impressive types of altered states involves feeling an invisible "presence". often interpreted as the awareness of god .Brain studies have found that this feeling comes about due to activity in an area of the temporal lobe. This " God Spot" is commonly activated in situations where a period of stress is suddenly brought to an end by a pleasant experience. It can also be stimulated artificially, or induced by transcranial magnetic stimulation (which inhabits activity in a specific part of the brain)

10 Altered States

At times the state of consciousness is altered slowly or suddenly. The change may be sudden and due to hallucinogenic drugs like LSD, a trance or religious ecstasy. It may be slow and indefinable. Some altered states are extraordinarily pleasant. Some spiritually oriented people or yogis experience a feeling of detachment from their own body and a sense of being fluid. There may also be a feeling of being bathed in bright light,or happiness of an extreme degree never experienced before and a profound sense of love and gratitude. It appears endless but lasts only for hours or days. The persons experiencing this are unaware and do not admit that these are illusions.

Neuroscientists say that these altered states occur when there is loss of normal coordination between different areas of the brain. In the normal state of consciousness, the neurons in different parts of the brain fire in synchrony and pool their information. This is achieved with the help of the neurotransmitter (hormone) dopamine. Dopamine is responsible for pleasure sensation. Simultaneously some neurotransmitters also oppose the action of dopamine and prevent total synchrony.

During peak phases of altered states, euphoria and seamlessness is observed. This is the result of hyper synchronization caused by

Altered states are caused by extreme psychological or physical stimuli such as drugs, chanting, dancing and flashing lights as well as by deep meditation.

combined effect of dopamine and serotonin.

Small changes in the oxygen balance of the brain can also affect consciousness. This is amply shown by the use of deep breathing techniques used for meditation. On the contrary, rapid, short breathing leads to the feeling of a fragmented world. The feelings of intense agitation and anxiety set in.

NDE

NDE is an altered state and a strange experience. It is dealt with in detail in a separate chapter.

Means of Achieving Altered States

Drugs

The altered states are either extremely pleasurable sensations or frightening. Drugs like LSD, cannabis ,heroin, ganja and marijuana are not new. Perhaps they are as old as civilization. They induce pleasure sensations easily and that is why these substances are addicting. The victims crave for them. It is difficult to give them up. These drugs act through chemical pathways in the brain – the increase in dopamine level. Some of these drugs affect serotonin and endorphin levels. Rise in these neurotransmitters leads to a feeling of serenity. Drugs like cocaine and amphetamines create a feeling of energy and power. These drugs act through an increased level of noradrenalin. Tranquillizers and anti-depressants act on specific brain cells producing predictable effects. They develop a habit in people to need higher doses for producing desired effects with habituation.

SomePhysical Activity

Altered states of consciousness can be obtained by better methods than drugs using sensory or psychological stimuli to alter brain activity through natural changes in the brain chemistry. Dancing with a rhythm and shutting off all other thoughts releases dopamine which is the pleasure hormone in the

Music can also produce such effects and can even lead to a further feeling of transcendence beyond pleasure, a spiritual experience.

limbic system. Dancers in this state can have out of body experiences. Osho used both dance and music to teach his disciples to achieve transcendence.

Meditation

Meditation is another way to achieve transcendence without drugs and rhythmic physical activities. Meditation can be achieved by focusing the mind on some thought, image, breathing or mantra. The objective of meditation is to get rid of all thoughts in the mind and create room for pure awareness. This is not an easy way. Scanning studies show that meditation reduces activities in the sensory cortex of the brain. Spiritual experience activates the temporal lobe of the brain which is also called the God Spot.

Hypnosis

Hypnosis has been defined as a special psychological state with certain physiological attributes superficially resembling sleep and marked by a functioning of the individual at a level of awareness other than the ordinary conscious state. Persons under hypnosis have heightened focus and concentration, with the ability to concentrate intensely on a specific thought or memory while blocking out sources of distraction. Hypnosis can be inducted by self suggestion (Self hypnosis), or by another persons suggestions. The hypnotic induction starts with eye fixation and suggestions and slowly person goes in hypnotic trance. The use of hypnotism for therapy is called hypnotherapy.

There is a belief that hypnosis is a form of unconsciousness resembling sleep but research suggests that hypnotized subjects are fully awake and are focusing their attention with a corresponding decrease in their peripheral awareness. The hypnotized person experiences heightened suggestibility and focus accompanied by a sense of tranquility and relaxation. The person sees, feels, smells and perceives all sensations in accordance with the suggestions of the hypnotist.

The common ailments in which hypnotherapy is used are: irritable bowel syndrome, pain management, warts, psoriasis and atopic dermatitis, and addiction to smoking. It is also used for reducing diet and stress. Medical science is not convinced of the therapeutic use of hypnotism beyond the use of suggestibility. However, surgeries have been done under hypnosis without anaesthesia.

The subconscious mind is a composite of everything one sees, hears or perceives as information. The mind collects information which it cannot otherwise consciously process to make meaningful sense. The conscious mind cannot always absorb disconnected information where it can be retrieved by the conscious mind when it needs to defend itself for survival or for solving puzzles. The subconscious mind stores information that the conscious mind may not immediately process with full understanding, but it stores the information for later retrieval when recalled by the conscious mind or a psychoanalyst. The subconscious mind instructing the conscious mind is called the inner thought or inner voice. This is often experienced in life-threatening situations. The subconscious mind is trying to guide the conscious because of the survival instinct. Techniques such as autosuggestion and affirmations are useful to harness the power of the subconscious to influence a persons life and outcomes of events in his daily life.

Hallucinations

Perception without a stimulus is hallucination. False perceptions are experienced by many of us in life. They may be in the form of heard footsteps on a dark night, the feeling of somebody putting a hand on our shoulder or figures seen in an empty corner of a dark room. They may be attributed the status of a ghost or god. If these experiences are mistaken for reality, they are called hallucinations. These are the sensory stimuli produced by our brain in the absence of any outside stimuli. These manufactured experiences are usually less vivid than real experiences based on actual external stimuli. This can happen in a normal brain or in a brain with altered functions because of drugs or illness. Spontaneous hallucinations are the result of an imaginary experience. This is often experienced in the twilight zones of sleep and waking.

Faith is the trigger. People who believe in ghosts see ghosts, people who believe in god, see God. The idols that are seen vary according to the different cultural and religious backgrounds. It is rightly said "The mind does not see what it does not know".

Hallucinations are common with drugs and sleep deprivation. Brain scans of subjects who hear hallucinating voices show that their auditory cortex is activated in just the same way as when the voices are actually heard. They also show that the voices are generated by the speech centers of the persons own brain.

Presupposition

Even when different persons see or perceive the same event and their sensory organs are giving the same inputs to their brains; still the perception of the event can vary with every individual. Those people who share a common culture, background and education are likely to perceive a similar event but people from different upbringing, education or cultural faiths will perceive it differently. If our religion and culture has taught us to kill certain animals and eat their meat, people from the same cult will find it in order. But if somebody from another culture believes in 'Ahimsa' and vegetarianism he finds this act cruel and unacceptable. Similarly mood swings can alter the interpretation of events. We experience such events in daily life though the events remain unchanged. They are also seen as reflections. A common example is that we become happy when we see our friend happy and gloomy when our dear one looks gloomy. The reason is believed to be the presence of mirror neurons in our brain.

Delusions

In patients suffering from schizophrenia, the perceptions seem to come from the real world but they are in fact hallucinations. Delusion is a set of fixed beliefs not amenable to reason and not shared by people of equivalent socio-cultural status. It is a disorder of thought. The sufferer feels as if they are real and internally generated. They can be dangerous at times.

Some Extraordinary Faculties of the Brain-

Imagination

Internally generated experiences are rarely as rich as those created by external stimuli because the brain is designed to give primary attention to the outside world. However, when we shut off the outside world by blindfolding or blocking our ears with a plug, there can be heightened imagination. This faculty is the source of artists which they use to enchant the world.

Intuition –

Intuition is another faculty of the brain which is beyond logic and possessed by rare people. When ideas and judgments surface unbidden to offer sudden insights into people and problems we call it an intuition. We cannot always rationalize these insights. Sometimes a person gets a sudden feeling that a dear one is in danger and later finds that it was really so. We intensely remember somebody and he/she contacts us. They call this telepathy. These are very personal experiences and cannot be proved scientifically or in a laboratory. They cannot be explained logically. We have to leave them as they are for the persons who experience them. As Shakespeares' Hamlet told Horatio

"There are more things in heaven and earth, Horatio, Than are dreamt of in your philosophy."

Déjà vu and Jamais vu

In life at times we have a feeling that we have experienced a thing earlier though we are actually experiencing it for the first time. It may be about a face or about a place. Usually, this feeling gives way soon and does not come back. Is this your mind tricking you in believing? Some people give it the color of re-incarnation.

Sigmund Freud thought that this is the floating of a repressed fantasy. This is thought to be a momentary lack of co-ordination between the two hemispheres of the brain. The latest view on this phenomenon is that this could be due to momentary lack of co-ordination between the cerebral cortex handling sensory information and the emotional pathways of the limbic system. 'Jama is Vu' is exactly opposite feeling. Here, if a person sees people or places he has seen before , instead of feeling familiar, he feels he is seeing them for the first time.. Such persons feel their usual surroundings and people are unfamiliar though they have been associated with them for a long time. This is attributed to temporary failure of the limbic system. This is seen progressively in diseases involving the limbic system. The sufferers often reject family members and may become paranoid and violent.

11 Learning

Learning means acquiring new knowledge or modifying or reinforcing existing knowledge. Learning is not the monopoly of human beings. Plants and animals also learn. They might have limited ways or means of learning. Man-made machines also learn and are likely to be intelligent in future.

There are different ways of learning whether intended / unintended formal or non-formal. The human brain starts learning to some extent in the womb of the mother. The process of learning becomes avid right from birth and continues throughout life.

Learning is an important activity of the brain in which memory plays a significant role. We memorise what we learn. Learning and memory are integral parts of each other.

Eyes, ears, nose, tongue and skin help us in learning. What we learn in school is imperative for a better quality of life in the long run. The learning after formal education is volitional. Observing and listening to others do help in learning but reading books and surfing on the internet are the best ways of updating our knowledge. One can never say that everything has been learnt.

The brain plays the highest and most crucial role in all the stages of learning. Fortunately, there is no limit for the capacity of the brain for learning, though at times there is a temporary feeling of exhaustion for a short while. Good sleep or a little diversion or relaxation can help rejuvenate the brain after which it is ready to take much more .

Human beings are blessed with a highly evolved brain, especially the neocortex. This gives them a distinct advantage in learning. It makes them intelligent and capable of using this learning ability to their advantage and for future guidance. We call this experience. High thinking power, imagination and emotions add to this advantage. This learning is a continuous process. Scientists have found evidence of behavioral learning as early as the 32nd week in intrauterine life. The development of the brain is very fast in foetal life. It continues at a rapid pace in the first two years after birth and is 85% complete till the age of 5. The fontanelle unite the suture joints of skull bones fuse . This puts severe limitations on the further quantitative growth of the brain. The neurons last almost for a life time; new neurons are not added except in a few small centers. The synaptic connections between the neurons however, can be added if the brain is provided stimulus. Thus, though nature limits learning, nurture can add to the learning and intelligence of the person. On the contrary, if you do not provide food, oxygen and exercise by way of an impetus for learning, transcranial the brain starts on a retrograde journey. This is why we call it –the use it or lose it principle. Man had a tail in the primordial stage but lost it because of disuse. Now only the tail bone remains. This is applicable to all the organs of the body in general and to the brain in particular.

The wider exposure and variety of knowledge provided to the next generation makes them smarter and intelligent. This is experienced by every generation. Even in the same generation we see that the younger sibling learns quicker than the elder one. This is because the younger one learns by observing and playing with the peer or elder one. This is factual and procedural knowledge. All the five sense organs contribute in learning. The next stage is the formal learning at school, learning through the teacher-student relationship.

Non-formal learning

International cultural exchange programmes are a good example of non-formal learning. They may also be in the form of workshops or training courses. It gives students a new insight in life to the student and helps them acquire new skills. It leads to mutual understanding among people of diverse cultures and from different geographies. Tangential learning is a way for self education, especially in a subject of our own interest. Self-education can be improved with systematic efforts.

Rote learning

The knowledge acquired out of school through different experiences and situations is informal learning. Rote learning is widely used in education for mastery over foundational knowledge. It is useful for quick memorization required for things such as learning one's lines in a play or lessons in an

> Rote learning is memorizing information by repetition. When the learnt knowledge is fully understood and used comprehensively in day-to-day context, it is called meaningful learning.

examination or memorizing telephone numbers. It is acquired by repetition or cramming. . Nowadays, children are encouraged more to research material for themselves than rote learning. This encourages better understanding and is retained in one's memory

Multimedia learning is audio-visual learning. Learning through computers and smart phone is e-learning. When we learn from an episode and use it for future guidance it is episodic learning. Semantic memory is the long term store of knowledge and facts.

Enculturation

This is a process in which a person learns the requirements of his native culture. He acquires the values, ideas, behavior, and rituals which are part of his surroundings. This is how we acquire our religion, thoughts, family and community values. Parents, other adults and peers contribute to this enculturation of an individual. Once rooted deeply, they are difficult to do away with. A person faces a cultural shock when he has to live in a society with a different culture. This is what leads to conflicts with other tribes or races. Learning to have a dialogue with others can help a lot in understanding their cultures.

Maturity and Creativity

Learning should not only be for passing examinations, getting degrees and money-making. It should give a person maturity. A person who has experience in life and can make use of a mature conscious mind can be called mature. Maturity is tested when a person has to make difficult decisions or resolve crises. Not all people mature fully. The degree of maturity depends on several factors such as age, cultural and moral background, opportunities for learning and the extent of exposure to the outer world.

A considered, constructive approach to problems and adjusting to changed circumstances with advancing age and experience are part of emotional maturity. People with emotional maturity will not be overdriven by achievements bogged down by temporary

Loud noises, suffocating atmosphere, stress and unnecessary intrusion from others lead to distraction and are counterproductive for creative, thoughtful and skilled tasks. Relaxing at regular intervals is an easy way to boost creativity in between tasks. Practice leads to perfection in performing tasks in a better way.

setbacks.

All of us have a desire to excel in whatever field we choose. The people who utilize their capacity, have a mind to think, and show commitment generally excel in their undertakings. They are able to create something not easily thought of by other people. . Techniques of meditation can help concentrate and be focused on the task. This is very useful for creativity.

Alertness

Our alertness is the alertness of the brain. A watchful, wide awake, brisk person is an alert person. Alertness of the mind can help us in completing our tasks. Here are some ways to make the brain alert.

Alertness depends on good sleep at night. All jobs needing skill are performed to the best of our ability if the mind is alert. It is observed that the colour yellow helps one to be alert.

Muscular activity, massage, optimal illumination of the work place, soothing music, a healthy and balanced diet and proper hydration are useful for alertness. The smell of citrus fruits create a stimulant effect on some people.

Alertness and drowsiness

Drowsiness and sleep are induced by serotonin. Serotonin is

synthesized from Gamma Amino Butyric Acid (GABA) in various parts of the brain. The reticular formation is a small part of the brain responsible for awareness, alertness, attention and concentration. GABA inhibits this center producing drowsiness and sleep. GABA is produced from an amino acid tryptophan. Milk is rich in tryptophan but most other foods are not.. When a person consumes a diet rich in carbohydrates (sweet, rice) , the hormone insulin is released by the pancreas. Insulin stimulates the uptake of 5 large alkaline amino acids into the muscle tissue leaving tryptophan in the blood. Thus as the relative level of tryptophan in the blood rises, more of it enters the brain. Thus GABA produces more serotonin which induces drowsiness and sleep following a high carbohydrate diet or consumption of milk.

Genius

A genius is a person whose brain has extraordinary and phenomenal capacity. Thomas Edison said :"Genius is 1% inspiration and 99% perspiration. "One gets creative ideas out of the blue and they often come in moments of relaxation or while idly toying with something else. But behind the ease of the creative flash lies the hard work that is always needed to bring the mind to the level of inspiration.

Wolf Girls and Tarzan

The following two stories suggest how the development of the brain and personality depends upon the kind of learning received by human beings. The brain of a newborn baby is fertile soil. If ,we sow healthy seeds rich in quality, we reap a healthy and fruitful crop. It is seen that the brain of a 14 week old foetus during gestation can perceive pain. All the same, we know that this is due to the primitive part of the brain and the evolved neocortex. The neurons in the neocortex are yet to be developed. This development starts soon after birth and then takes up a phenomenal pace. The growth of neurons at birth is quarter of a million per minute. The synaptic connections also develop at a brisk rate. The growth of neurons in most of the areas except a few is almost complete by the age of two years but the synaptic connections continue to grow till the age of 30 years. All the sensory organs start giving inputs (sowing seeds) soon after birth. This is the beginning of learning. The matter learnt is encoded and stored into memory. Memory is revisited and revised with every piece of new and perceived knowledge . This is what we call experience. Development of the mind, unconscious and conscious, is a sum of all such experiences. Children learn very fast and develop their speech and vocabulary. Organs or faculties develop in the proportion to the use made of them on the principle - use it or lose it. Use more and have more.

If the child is deprived of any source of learning up to the age of 5 years, it is less likely to learn easily in later years of life. Let it be walking, talking or body language. This is amply demonstrated by the example of wolf girls.

It is the story of two sisters, Amala and Kamala. The names were given to them by a missionary who rescued them from wolves in 1920. It seems these two girls were left or got lost in a jungle. They were nurtured by wolves in the jungle. As the girls were fostered and brought up by wolves, they could not speak or understand human language. They could make noises like wolves, walked and ran on four limbs, ate raw meat, showed no facial expressions and preferred the company of the dogs of the missionary. Their hearing and eyesight were very sharp like wolves. This example demonstrates the importance of surroundings that influence our learning of speech, facial expression, body language and development of various human faculties.

Tarzan, the ape man is a fictitious character created by Edgar Rice Burroughs but suggests the same principle. Tarzan imitated the apes who nurtured him and his surroundings made him what he was.

12 Memory - The Treasure

The memory of human beings is a unique gift of nature to them. Probably animals and plants have very little of it as compared to human beings. Memory is a process of retaining, storing and retrieving impressions or things learnt in the past. All the five important sense organs are receiving information constantly and fixing it in the store house known as the brain. This information is recalled whenever needed. There is no particular centre or geographical area of the brain solely responsible for this job. It is a well coordinated effort of multiple parts of the brain as a whole. The reassembly of all the events in the past creates a new version in the light of any new experiences or information for present and future guidance. It is not only a recall of old learning.

Memory is not a single-handed function. It involves recognition as well as recalling of stored information. Recognition is comparatively easy and quick particularly when a place or human faces are revisited, While recalling involves more stages of memory processing, if it is a large piece of information.

Memory begins with the first breath and gives us company till the last gasp. It functions throughout our life .

This is in part a gift of nature that is determined by the genes and can be improved upon by efforts. Various techniques are used for this purpose.

The information received from the sense organs in the form of chemical and physical stimuli is encoded and then stored by this faculty. It is recalled, whenever required, to assess the information received in a new context. A new, overall revised concept, is formed, encoded again and stored afresh for use now and in future. Some recalls are effortless while other need some effort.

Like any other human ability, memory is also fallible. In spite of its limitless capacity, what we recall or use is just a fraction of the vast store of information in our memory. The ability to memorize is both, a gift of nature received through our genes and an achievement through nurture and efforts such as techniques and practice.

Memory and Identity

Positive and negative experiences of the past, perceptions of events and emotions shape our identity. Every individual's memory is his private library. An autobiographical memory is by and large the result of our own inner record and inner myths. Childhood memories are cherished by most individuals. Of course, very little long term memories are formed before the age of four.

Identity Disorders

We read books and watch movies about crimes with interest. Some texts depict crimes committed by people whose psychiatrist claims that his client is a victim of multiple personality disorder.

Yes! There are some people who are really the victims of personal identity disorders. A search by (through) psychoanalysis leads us to the root cause. Quite often the cause is physical and sexual abuse of the victim in childhood. The pain and horror of the abuse divides the persons memory in splinters and stores it in different parts (of the brain) splitting his/her personality. Thus deep rooted splits lead to alternative personalities sharing the same brain.

Hypno-therapy is suggested by some psychotherapists for multiple personality disorders but has not been uniformly useful.

Memory and Intelligence

Memory and intelligence do not necessarily go hand in hand. A person may be very intelligent but without very good memory and vice versa but there is some connection between memory, skill and talent or mental performance. Intelligence works for physical activities and logical mathematical, linguistic, social and musical skills. Sensory memory is formed mainly in three ways. Iconic memory, based on visual information which decays fast, echoic memory, from auditory signals and the memory sourced by touch sensation which is called the haptic memory.

Memory and Gender

It seems that males and females have some differences in memory, skills, which are attributed to hormonal differences. The right and left brain pathways have a slight difference. The left brain specializes in processing detailed

Cultures have collective memories. Every culture in the world has some collective memories of its own. Idols, images, ideas particularly related to god, deities, mythologies and religions are the examples of the age-old collective memories.

information. Women tend to use this more, that is why they are better than men at details. They are faster in "spotting the difference" than men. They are more accurate in recognizing plants. Men use the right brain more which gives them slight advantage in spatial memory such as reading maps of locations. Women can recall and read faces better. The testosterone inhibits left brain processing while estrogen boosts it. These memory differences are certainly very small compared to the individual differences acquired through genes, nature, training and nurture. We remember better when we are attentive and we dont if we are stressed or inattentive.

Capacity of Memory

When we say, "I cannot take it anymore", it means we are not in a receptive mood and not that the capacity of the brain is exhausted. The capacity of the brain is   limitless. There is a limit to the number of neurons but not to the synaptic connections between the neurons. Memory is the function of increasing the synaptic connections which has no limits.

Experiences become memories because the neurons produce them from/through connections with one another. Each time an event is recalled the neural firing pattern is changed slightly. This new memory overwrites the old one. In short, new memories are a modification of earlier memories and not merely recollections of events from the past. Thus, there can be infinite versions of early memory. However clear the memory may seem, it is rarely a precise match with the actual event which is experienced.

This is called enculturation. In the days before the art of writing and recording, these memories were transferred from one generation to another by storytellers, clerics and leaders of societies. Most of this knowledge was in oral forms like poems, mythological stories, fairytales or folktales. This was a sort of historical tradition of a community. More permanent records came in the form of cave paintings, manuscripts on papyrus which was a paper prepared from plants and today we have wonderful audio and video recordings.

Good Memory A Gift or Earned Skill

Good memory-call it a gift of nature or a genetic gift- exists from birth without any of the techniques or methods used to remember things. This gift may be all inclusive or for a special kind of memory task. Some persons are blessed with exceptional mathematical abilities. An examples Shakuntala Devi, from India who could do multiplication of multiple digit numbers within a moment. People took longer time to verify it using the computer. Mozart could not only repeat music composed by somebody else with some effort at the age of 14 but could also improve upon it. Such talent is found in some normal individuals as well as some autistic children (2%). On one hand these children qualify to be called idiots but when they exhibit such extraordinary skill they are called "Idiot Savants."

Some people not gifted with such abilities can supersede normal and average people in some tasks related to the memory by using techniques for remembering. If a person with inborn talent also practices these techniques of linking words, numbers or pictures interchangeably, they can exhibit great memory skills. At the same time some of these gifted people are found lacking in general ability though they are exceedingly well in one(particular) memory skill. The education system should spot such students and give them special attention. They should be groomed and encouraged to use their skill for the good of the nation.

Photographic Memory

The technique of photography was developed in the 19th century and it has made phenomenal progress since then. Scientists doing research on photographic memory have failed to find a memory which can give details in the same manner as when one sees and describes a scene. However, some young children have a limited form of photographic memory. They have an ability to hold strong visual images in their mind. This is called eidetic memory but it fades as they grow up.

Types of Memory

Short term memory

Short term memory is also called working memory. This lasts from a few seconds to a minute. It is compared to the writing on a blackboard. It is just like jotting a point, wiping it clean after a short time and then starting to write new things. It is also called a sketchpad. Similarly, there is a short-term phonological record as well. Both of these use different areas of brain. The sensory memory and short term memory generally have a strictly limited capacity and duration. Short term memory is supported by transient patterns of neuronal communications and encodes the information acoustically or iconically in the temporal lobe, parietal lobe and occipital lobes.

Long term memory

Memory stored from hours to years is long term memory. It can store enormous amount of information for a potentially unlimited period or even a whole life. Long term memory encodes semantically. It is maintained by the more stable and permanent changes in neural connections widely spread throughout the brain. Hippocampus plays an important role in converting short-term memory to long term memory. One of the important functions of sleep is consolidation of information through rehearsal.

Every time a particular set of neurons fire together, it becomes more likely that they will fire together in future. When such connections are repeatedly activated by rehearsal, they form links which last even more, making them a single unit. This is important for long term memory. Iconic memory formed by visual impressions tends to fade earlier than echoic memory formed by hearing. Memory for skills and events is encoded in long term memory.

Biased Memories

Memories formed by us are not a simple record of experience. In fact they are the biased reconstructions of what is learnt. They are all influenced by our personal habits of the mind, prejudices and preconceptions of events experienced. People find it easier to remember what they already believe than the information that challenges their existing ideas. Memory stores things that seem important at the moment of experience and selectively preserves those memories favorable or suitable to us. Memory is constructed actively by the brain and it is not merely a passive process.

Procedural Memories –

When earlier experiences affect our bias, thinking and behavior without awareness it is called implicit memory. Resemblance triggers good or bad feelings for a person in the very first meeting. An interesting observation is that chewing gum may have a beneficial effect on memory. This is seen in an f-MRI scan. It could be that the pleasurable sensation reduces the level of stress hormone (cortisol) in the hippocampal cells. People with amnesia also preserve procedural memories.

Relation Of Senses And Memory

Memories formed by different sense organs have something special and common in them.

Visual Memory

Our visual center is situated in the occipital lobe. It is said that pictures or paintings speak volumes when written words fall short of description. Information can be stored well by innumerable visual impressions. Our memory for images remains fantastic all through out our lives. If we try, we can recreate vivid details of a scene from our visual memory as if it were photographic library. This is well demonstrated in the forensic field. Artists prepare the sketches of criminals on the basis of description from the witness. If witnesses are taken to the scene of accident or crime, they can recollect the incident better. It is also seen that students fare better in examinations if they are seated in the classroom where they have learnt than in some other place. Different chemicals (neurotransmitters) are associated with emotions: acetylcholine with excitement, dopamine with pleasure and glutamate with disgust. We say - birds of the same feather flock together. This applies to emotional memories. They are better recalled in an emotional state. These are context-related memories which become hooked up by association.

Echoic Memory

Specialized memory is formed for sounds and music. The center for hearing is situated in the temporal lobe. Wernickes area in the temporal lobe responds to speech while those on the right temporal lobe register melody and tone. Cells in the limbic system produce an emotional reaction to sounds creating fear or delight.

Echoic memory helps a car mechanic or a doctor to diagnose a problem of the car engine or human machine.

Taste and Touch Memories

Touch and taste also contribute to recall episodic memory. If more than one sensory organ has contributed to a particular episodic memory or emotion, it is more easily recalled by the brain. This is like putting more men on the job to finish it quickly

Scents (smells) and Memory

It is well known that different kinds of smells are very potent in triggering memories of the past. There is a strong link between smell, episodic memory and emotions. This episodic memory is stored in the amygdala hippocampal complex, which is developed from the olfactory system.

Memories of Emotions

Memories associated with emotional episodes are recalled easily. The more powerful the emotions, the quicker the recollection of the episode. This is because we pay more attention to the emotional episodes and attention is the first stage of laying down a memory. Unattractive facts are also memorized if presented immediately after watching an emotionally moving film.

Ways to Enhance Memory

Sometimes we struggle to retrieve something. This is temporary loss of a particular memory. Once memory is formed and stored in the form of long-term memory, there can be a temporary problem in retrieval. Then we say, "It is on the tip of my tongue but is not coming out." We are tongue-tied. We make efforts. We search for clues – "It starts with the letter "C". It has 3 or 4 letters in it. It is not this. I know it but it is not coming to my mind. I mean .... ", and all of a sudden like a flash the right word comes. If it does not happen, we should switch our attention to something else or try to keep other words that come to us away. We should use the free associations method (given by psycho-analysts like Sigmund Freud) of the word, re-establish the context for the episode or the best way is to sleep on it or try to relax. The answer will come in a dream or after sleep.

Everybody wants to possess a good memory and newspapers are full of attractive advertisements of various medicines which guarantee an increase in the strength of our memory.

Here are some ways of doing that without spending money on medicines.

a) Chunking information is one way. If we want to remember lengthy telephone numbers, it is useful to break them in groups of three or four and to give names to groups of numbers familiar to us. Children remember the 26 English alphabets in groups by using rhymes or rhythms. Memories associated with emotional and pleasurable events are easily encoded in long term memory. Procedural memories or procedural memory skills like swimming or driving are stored in long term memory and are permanent. Unpleasant memories and those used sparsely tend to be lost soon. People with amnesia also preserve procedural memories. When earlier experiences affect or show a bias in our thinking and behavior without awareness, it is called implicit memory. Resemblance triggers good or bad feelings for a person in the very first meeting.

Good Memory for Children and Students

Newborns develop memories about the touch and smell of the mother but the episodic memories are neither formed nor recalled up till the age of three. This is the period when the brain is still maturing. Gradually, repetition of the learning experience starts forming long term memory. Teenagers become aware of their physical and mental strengths and limitations. This is the time when they become selective in acquiring skills and developing interests in subjects they like. In adulthood, they start learning skills for their chosen career. Even after retirement learning does not stop. They learn to adapt to the leisurely life, hobbies and traveling. At this age memory doesn't fail but is certainly slowed down because of changes due to aging and can fail further because of trauma or disease. Students learn by rote learning (repetition or cramming). Project work makes them more creative and technological aids like audio-visuals and computers are very useful. Studies done at a quiet place help in concentration, and such an ambience helps in remembering things in a better way. Sleeping immediately after studies helps in rehearsals during REM sleep which makes the memory long lasting. Distractions during or after studies and physical and mental stress prove to be counter-productive in learning.

If learning of a subject is done with understanding, it is better retained. Repetition after short intervals is helpful. One of the effective ways of improving memory of written material is the PQRST method.

P – preview, Q – question, R – read, S – self recitation and T - test.

While preparing for examinations or speeches students should jot down points and also try to use mnemonics such as number and shape methods, rhymes, and peg systems. One more technique used for remembering the learnt information is to tag it with some predetermined number, peg, picture or an easy-to-remember sentence and then to visualize the tags with the information tagged on them. It becomes easy to recall the information.

A diet rich in complex carbohydrates such as bread, rice,

vitamins and minerals is ideal for maintaining a good memory. Alcohol, tobacco and caffeine must be avoided.

Eating too much diverts more blood to the digestive system and reduces blood supply to the brain. This reduces the memory function and one feels sleepy. Similarly, when a student is hungry, the blood sugar level goes down and the brain cannot function efficiently. It is advisable to have small meals 3-4 times a day and avoid overeating as well as undereating.

Care for Memory

What must we do to care for our memory? We have to maintain good physical and mental health. This is achieved by a good diet, physical exercise and good sound sleep. We must avoid excess stress. Moderate amount of stress is positive and it gives us a sense of responsibility and urgency which makes us attentive. This is productive. Rewards and punishment affect the memory. By thinking young we, can be better in memory tasks like the youth. Even if we retire from work, we must keep ourselves busy in hobbies, arts and games like chess or bridge and solve puzzles. Use the brain and you will never lose it.

Herbal Remedies –

Sage (Salvia officinals) oil reduces the effect of the enzyme cholinesterase. This helps maintain the level of a neurotransmitter acetylcholine which is useful in developing memory. Eggs, cabbage and caviar. Vitamin B complex in general and B 1 in particular are useful for memory. Green vegetables, fish, chicken, oatmeal and whole grains help the memory perform better. Vitamins in fruits, vegetables and food are very useful for memory. A vitamin supplement is needed only if there is a deficiency. Taking caffeine in moderate quantities of coffee, tea and colas helps in increasing alertness, but it is wrong to say that it increases brain function or memory. In fact, excess quantities of caffeine affect the functioning of the brain adversely.

Sleep and Memory

The relationship of sleep and memory are cordial and intimate. We always want to avoid memories of unpleasant episodes. When we learn about an event or a subject of study before going to sleep, the brain does not sleep completely. It is not taking complete rest. In fact it is busy revising the events and the knowledge acquired before sleep. This occurs in the rapid eye movement (REM) sleep. This is how the brain encodes and fixes the acquired knowledge in the long term memory. This is the reason why students must make sure of good sleep after reading or studying. Exercise, particularly aerobics, running, cycling and swimming have cognitive benefits on the brain. This is because of improved levels of oxygen, nutrients neurotransmitters and increased neurogenes is in the hippocampus. This helps children in academics, maintaining mental abilities in old age and is also a potential cure for neurological diseases.

Scientists have been working and researching on the phenomenon of memory. The article "Electrical Current to boost memory" in SCI-Tech, Pune Mirror – Sep. 3 2014 adds to our knowledge about memory. Scientists have succeeded in improving memory impaired by trauma or disease by Tran-cranial Magnetic Stimulation (TMS). This is a technique that involves non-invasive delivery of electrical currents using magnetic impulses. This is being tried on patients suffering from stroke, early-stages of Alzheimer's disease, traumatic brain injury, cardiac arrest leading to hypoxia of brain and memory problems caused by healthy aging. Scientists have achieved encouraging results in these cases through use of TMS. This non-invasive stimulation improves the ability to learn new things. It has tremendous potential for treating memory disorders.

The Northwestern Medicine Study has also demonstrated that remembering events requires a collective effort and co-relation of many areas of the brain with the hippocampus. An electrical stimulation is like giving the brain region a more talented conductor for the task of memory.

TMS continues to improve memory up to 24 hours after the stimulus.

A person with brain damage or a memory disorder benefits from this technique because their neural networks are disrupted. In case of a person with a normal memory and the brain working effectively, however, there will be no added advantage.

The scientist Vosswho has been researching TMS cautions that years of research are needed to determine whether this approach is safe or effective for patients with Alzheimer's disease or similar memory disorders.

Another article "Memory Manipulations?" in the 'Times of India-30 Aug 2014—pg12] also tells us about some other findings in this field. Everybody has some memories that they cherish and some that hurt. When sad memories become ugly it shows in the form of psychiatric disorders. Research in manipulating memory by neuroscientists at MIT in the US can prove helpful to those millions across the globe who lead miserable lives on account of bad experiences stored in their memory. Manipulating these unwanted memories is an effective way of transforming the lives of this unfortunate lot. Incase it works to address such negative experiences through stored memory it will surely be worth it.

Prof. Susumu Tonegava, a neuroscientist at MIT, US says that memories per say are neutral. They are not pleasant or unpleasant. The emotions or feelings created by certain groups of memories are cherished while other groups create unpleasant emotions of extreme degree and are responsible for psychiatric disorders. In a normal person a mix of both types of emotions is conducive to a healthy life.

Idiot Savants (autistics)

2% of autistics have some exceptional skill or ability. In the autistic brain, most of the brain modules are damaged, but there is a cortical island that is spared. This island spontaneously allocates all the attentional resources to the one module that's still functioning in the parietal lobe. Thus this becomes hyper functioning giving extraordinary skill or talents.

13 Forget It!

Something about FORGETTING

Forgetting is not an active process by itself. It is a lapse at some stage when memory is being formed. In fact, if some information is received at a time when the brain is pre-occupied in some other task, the memory is not formed at all though the brain has been given the inputs. The brain then fails to register. Once the inputs have been accepted, they are classified. The brain does not like to recall unpleasant memories to the extent possible. of. It would like to keep them from surfacing.

A common dictum in medicine is "use it or lose it". Memory and other functions of the brain follow this golden rule. In the course of time, items that are rarely used degrade or become over written by new thoughts and ideas. Disease and trauma to the brain can cause permanent memory loss. Similarly, advancing age, lack of exercise or narrowing of the blood vessels of the brain cause degenerative changes of the brain. This

> If the human brain has unlimited capacity for memory, why do we forget? Nobody can boast that he or she remembers everything. Everybody forgets. There may be a difference only of degree.

happens in all the organs of the body. The brain also shrinks in size. This inevitably leads to decreased ability of its overall functions. Memory is no exception. However, if blood circulation to the brain is sufficient if the person takes regular physical exercise and uses his brain for memory tasks, his memory may remain in an excellent condition in spite of physical aging.

Forgetting is also a part of the game. We cannot remember everything. Anyone can forget irrespective of age. But age-related changes usually contribute more to forgetfulness. Our ability to recognize information which has been previously   is largely unaffected by age. But recalling of names may require more effort. Often elderly people cannot recall names (nominal alphasia) easily,(the tip of tongue phenomenon). However, procedural memory verbal memory, unconscious memory and expertise largely remain unaffected.

Eye Witness Testimony

When a person sees things with his own eyes, he thinks he will remember them well. If he is standing in court as an eye witness, he is convinced that what he is testifying in the court of law is true. Yet, during cross-examination he can be made to contradict his statement through suggestions which can confuse him. This makes an eyewitness unreliable. Children are more prone to such confusions of suggestibility. Many legal cases rely heavily on eyewitnesses. A study in the US has shown that 4500 false or wrong convictions were made in a single year.

Decay of memory – Amnesia - Dementia - Alzheimers Dementia

Forgetting is human, so we may not bother much about it. However, forgetting takes a grave form in the diseases related to memory disorders like Amnesia dementia and Alzheimer's dementia.

Researchers are divided on the subject. Some researchers say that memories simply decay while others are of the opinion that new memories disrupt them.

Herman Ebbinghaus, a German Psychologist found that after reading some lists of nonsense syllables(consisting of a sequence of consonant vowel and consonant) the forgetting occurred most rapidly at the beginning. Subsequently, however, forgetting happened at a slower rate. This happens if we simply store information without rehearsing or refreshing the knowledge. There may be interference due to old memories (retroactive) or new information (proactive). Both contribute to forgetting.

Amnesia is a temporary or permanent impairment in the formation or retrieval of memory, while dementia is a category of brain diseases which involves the loss of ability to think and reason clearly. This can affect daily activities of an individual. Amnesia progresses with age. Delirium is an acute, reversible mental disorder characterized by confusion and some impairment of consciousness. It is generally associated with emotional liability, hallucinations and delusions. Delirium may be a secondary symptom of some diseases of the brain. High fever, encephalitis, meningitis and metabolic disorders also cause delirium.

Amnesia can be due to brain damage due to trauma, infection or degenerative disease. When the temporal lobe is affected, it contributes to memory loss. Amnesia following trauma can last for hours, days or months but complete recovery is possible. Alzheimers disease and stroke lead to lasting or permanent amnesia. If amnesia is regarding some event in the past it is termed retrograde amnesia. The victims can forget who they are and what their past was. However our memory for tasks like driving, reading and other skills is relatively resistant to amnesia. The victims can also learn new skills. This is because different parts of the brain viz. cerebellum and putamen are involved in the skills.

Amnesia is the loss of memory in part or in full. This usually follows damage to the brain by physical trauma, disease or psychological trauma. Sedatives and hypnotic drugs can produce it temporarily. Amnesia is of two types. Retrograde amnesia occurs when one cannot remember events before the accidental trauma. It may be for a period of months or many years. It is as if a key to the store of past memory is lost. Anterograde amnesia is amnesia where an accident leads to problems in transferring new information to the memory from the day of the damage. Damage to the medial temporal lobe or the hippocampus can cause this.

In anterograde amnesia, the memory loss is due to the lack of ability to store new information in the memory. This happens gradually like in Alzheimer's or chronic alcohol abuse (Korsakoffs syndrome). Damage to or surgical removal of the hippocampus is another cause of anterograde amnesia. Generally when amnesia is in a progressive or permanent state the brain can retrieve part of the ability of storing memory by newly formed paths or synaptic connections.

Dementia is a mental disorder which results in impairment in intellectual functioning frequently characterized by failing memory, difficulty in calculating, distractibility, mood swings, and leads to judgment and orientation being affected. Dementia is generally irreversible, unless it is due to some other disease which is curable.

Alzheimers affects aged persons and it progresses with age. There is no cure for this disease. It worsens as age advances and eventually leads to death. Alzheimers usually starts after the age of 65 years. Incase it occurs earlier it is called early onset A. D. Thirteen percent of the cases of early onset AD are familial, where a genetic predisposition is seen.

The suffering starts with impairment of learning and memory, difficulty with language and execution of movements. Recent memories are lost first and the older ones later. Wandering, irritability, aggression, illusions, delusions, urinary incontinence, apathy, exhaustion, reduction in muscle mass, pressure, ulcers and pneumonia are the terminal events caused by Alzheimers.

Clinical Picture

Different kinds of pictures may be seen in different people. The common symptoms are stress, short term memory loss and reduced thinking abilities. As the disease worsens, confusion, irritability, aggression, mood swings and then long term memory loss set in.

The C.T. scan of the brain shows marked shrinkage. The life expectancy of the patients is seven years. Only 3% survive for fourteen years.

No cure is possible but a balanced diet, physical, exercise and mental stimulation exercises can delay the onset of the disease. This is a neurodegenerative disorder. The person becomes dependent on others. This puts a lot of social, psychological, physical and economic strain on the patient and his family.

The exact cause of AD is not known. There are many different views. One thing is certain that it is a degenerative disorder characterized by loss of neurons and synapses in the cerebral cortex and some other areas.

One way of prevention is by engaging in intellectual activities, reading, writing board games, playing music which may delay AD.

The discussion of memory and forgetting should help enhance our understanding of memory. Of course, it is necessary to remember our duties towards others such as our family, society and country etc. But do remember one thing - it is always nice to forget some things in life, for instance faults of others, wrongs done to us, our help to others and so on. Forgive and forget – this is the golden rule of life.

Spatial Memory

Dr. John O Keef has been awarded the Nobel prize in Medicine (Oct. 2014), for his research about space cells and grid cells in the hippocampus. These are the neurones specialising in the memory of place and orientation. When the function of these cells is disturbed in head injuries or disease, the patient loses orientation of time and place. They ask questions like, where am I? Who am I and so on? This may be a temporary phase during recovery. This research may bring some solace to victims of Alzheimer's disease who loose these sensations due to degenerative changes in the brain.

14 Sleep

Sleep is certainly one of the fundamental needs of life and neuroscientists stress that it is necessary for survival. We can somehow manage to live without food for 10-15 days but we cannot survive that long without sleep. This is the reason why prisoners of war or spies are not allowed to sleep. Thus, the task of getting them to tell their deeply and deliberately guarded secrets becomes easy.

Poets equate sleep with sweet rest for the mind and soul. Shakespeare suggests in his plays that a person with a guilty conscience cannot sleep well. In his famous drama Macbeth, Lady Macbeth instigates her husband Macbeth to murder King Duncan so that he would become the King and she the Queen. She becomes the Queen but loses her sleep. Every night she walks in her sleep, sees blood stains on her hands and keeps washing them, and at last commits

> People normally think that the brain is taking rest during sleep. Contrary to this, the brain is very busy when the person is sleeping. It is learning continuously when the person is awake. Everything that is happening around is taken note of, whether consciously or unconsciously, by the brain.

suicide.

The work of storing the information in the short term or long term memory is done by the brain after the information is received. This needs revision, classification, storage or rejection and sleep is the best time for the brain to accomplish this task. No new information is being received by the brain during this time. This prevents interference in its work. This may be comparable to the ruminating of animals by bringing what has been eaten to the mouth from the stomach at leisure and at will. Pandit Jawaharlal Nehru used to say "Change of work is rest". Human brain has known this since the inception of humanity.

A common man experiences the importance of sleep only when deprived of it for a few days. The requirement of sleep can vary according to the individual needs. Age, exercise, tension, anxiety, fatigue and the environment all modify the requirements of sleep. Infants and children need more sleep. This is conducive for physical and mental growth at that age. A normal adult needs good sound sleep for 6-8 hours and this requirement goes on reducing as age advances.

Sleep has a rhythm in normal people. It is called circadian rhythm. This is called the clock in the brain. The smallest identifiable part of the brain, the pineal body, is responsible for this rhythm. It secretes a hormone: Melatonin. When light is shut off by closing the eyes and this secretion of Melatonin is reduced and the person awakes when daylight appears. Everybody can manage to get up early if the need for sleep has been met with or with an alarm. Yet, it can happen even when one is not using an alarm because the mind reminds us of important assignments like catching a midnight flight or an emergency phone call. Thus an order is followed.

However, there can be disorder of sleep as well. When we are unable to sleep in spite of need for it we call it "Insomnia"

Primary Insomnia -

If the sleeplessness occurs independently of any known physical or mental abnormality, it is called Primary Insomnia. The person may have difficulty in falling asleep or may wake up frequently. If this happens continuously for at least a month, it is a sign of this disorder.

Remedy

The remedial measures can be:

a)To follow your sleep routine and reduce the time spent in bed during the day.

b)Discontinuing drugs like Caffeine, Nicotine, and Alcohol.

c)Avoid taking naps at odd times.

d)Follow a physical fitness regimen.

e) Avoid listening to radio, watching television and taking a hot shower before going to bed.

e)Eating at regular times and avoiding over-eating.

f)Practicing relaxation of muscles and meditation.

g) Maintaining a comfortable bed room and bed.

If these non-specific measures do not work, consult your doctor and take medicines for a short period.

Primary Hypersomnia –

When there is excessive sleep without a known physical or mental disorder it is Primary hypersomnia. If it persists for more than a month, stimulants like Amphetamine can be given in the morning to treat it.

Sleep Apnea

Snoring during sleep is a common. All voluntary muscles relax during sleep. In some people the tongue falls back and obstructs the air passage with deep relaxation through the oral route and a similar relaxation of the muscles of the uvula leads to obstruction of the nasal route. Thus, due to the entire route being blocked, entry of air into the lungs is obstructed and oxygenation of the blood is reduced. This causes deprivation of oxygen to the all important brain. This can happen for intervals of 10-20 seconds sometimes longer and about five hundred times every night.

Oxygen starvation of the brain for 3-4 minutes can cause irreversible damage to the brain or even death. Persons suffering from sleep apnea have severe morning headaches in the morning, confusion, depression, anxiety and much physical fatigue. High blood pressure, irregular heartbeats and heart failure occur if the apnea is neglected for long.

Treatment

a) If the patient is obese, he should reduce weight and avoid all sorts of sedatives like alcohol and nicotine.

b) He should sleep on one side and not on his back to the extent possible.

Some more dos are - Reduce pillows and raise the head end of the bed by 300. If these measures fail, sleep studies like polysomnography must be done. Some patients benefit from surgery of the throat. Positive pressure ventilation devices also help some of these victims. In 84% of the patients the cause is peripheral and local. They are likely to benefit from these measures. In 0.4% of the patients the cause for apnea is a central one. The brain forgets to give orders to breathe and such patients can succumb to apnea. In 15% of patients the cause is combined - central and peripheral.

Pace Makers

For those having a central or a mixed cause, a pacemaker may be needed to stimulate the phrenic nerve (diaphragm). This remedy is still in an experimental stage. It works on the same principle as the pacemaker of the heart.

Parasomnia

There are other sleep disorders like nightmares, sleep walking, and bruxism. Sexomania is another sleep disorder in which the person engages in a sexual act while still asleep. The person can even rape during this phase. This happens if he comes in physical contact with a person in bed. The psychiatrist can study the history of the patient and opine about it in criminal defense if he is convinced about the act having been done during sleep. The person doing it does not remember it when he wakes up.

Sleep disorders secondary to other physical or mental disorders need careful assessment and treatment by the physician.

Sleep and Dreams

Sleep and dreams are altered states of consciousness in day-to-day life. Sleep is a physiological process absolutely essential for life. All the organs in the body including the brain are taking rest to the extent possible. It gives them time to recover lost energy and regenerate lost cells as much as possible.

Sleep is a temporary transition where consciousness is partially shut off. The brain is still active and the sleeping person can awaken easily. Studies on sleep show that it consists of two parts:

Slow Wave Sleep or SWS and Rapid Eye Movement sleep or REM.

We start with SWS and alternate it with REM, so called because the eye balls are making rapid movements during this phase of sleep. Mental activity is at the lowest ebb during SWS but most of the dreaming is experienced during the REM phase. These dreams are far from reality. The less frequent dreams in the SWS are termed drowsy thoughts and they are not bright images. These are like real life experiences. SWS is essential for maintenance of health and growth.

In REM sleep, brain activity in the brainstem is inhibited. The voluntary muscles are relaxed as if temporarily paralyzed. This helps us like a safety mechanism. We do not act physically in dream experiences. During REM sleep the brain is busy rehearsing the knowledge obtained during waking state. That is why it is recommended that students must have good sleep after reading so that the matter learnt is processed and stored in their long term memory.

People used to claim that they can diagnose and cure diseases or predict future events by analyzing dreams. This has no rationale. The legendary psychoanalyst Sigmund Freud put forth a theory in his book "Interpretation of Dreams" that unfulfilled desires and expectations, particularly sexual desires are expressed in dreams. He cured many patients using interpretations of dreams and counseling on the basis of psychoanalysis.

Interpretation of dreams has been an interesting subject for centuries. Every culture has a large treasure of stories and superstitions about dreams.

Day dreaming is another interesting subject. The person dreaming during the awakened state is usually either ambitious like successful Bollywood stars or lazy like any average person. These ambitions are based on conscious thinking. Many times such dreaming makes them focused and hard working. It often helps them achieve their goals partially or fully. a man was lost in lazy day dreaming about getting enormous wealth by selling his pitchers, then marrying a pretty girl and some day kicking her if she disobeyed him. While kicking her in his dream, he kicked the earthen pitchers and broke them and along with them his dreams.

Day dreaming is a short term detachment from ones immediate surroundings during which a person's contact with reality is blurred and partially substituted by a visionary fantasy. Sometimes it gives people happy, pleasant thoughts or fulfillment of hopes or ambitions.

Lucid Dreams

Lucid dreaming is any dream in which one is aware that one is dreaming. In common dreams experienced during REM sleep, we are passive observers and we have no conscious control on the dream. Lucid dreams are rational, there is a clear perception and we understand the meaning. We are allowed to control the dreams but there is no constraint on physical laws. You can fly like a bird, chat to your dear ones or stroll in the garden. In these dreams the brain's control centre wakes up and restores the sense of self. Lucid dreams can occur spontaneously but some people can train themselves to have such lucid dreams by visualizing techniques.

15 Mind's Drama

We play games for physical and mental health or for the joy we get out of them. The mind however, plays games for other reasons also.

Malingering

Malingering is fabricating or exaggerating the symptoms of mental or physical disorders for some gain. It may be for financial gain, it may be avoiding work or school, obtaining drugs to which the person is addicted, to avoid punishment or to gain sympathy.

Malingerers show physical or psychological symptoms in order to accomplish specific goals. They have many vague or poorly localized complaints which are presented in great detail. They get irritated if the doctor is skeptical about their history. A good clinician can easily find out if the person is feigning or malingering.

If the results of physical examination and lab tests are negative, no medical treatment is required. The patient should be encouraged to ventilate his feelings. A good clinician should identify the areas of secondary pain and help the person manage his stress. Gradually the patient will give up (stop showing) the symptoms. Malingering is more common in men of working age than women.

In the 19th century, hysteria was a common diagnosis predominant among women. In these cases psychological problems were transformed into dramatic physical symptoms. Well known psychiatrist, Sigmund Freud was of the opinion that all these problems are rooted in the suppression of sexual desires right from infancy. This theory is controversial.

Conversion Reaction

The term hysteria is hardly used by the doctors now. Freud's basic ideas of physical symptoms caused by unconscious conflict or pain remain unchanged though the tag of sexual reason is not accepted by all.

> Conversion Reaction is defined as the appearance of symptoms affecting the movements or the senses which are hard to explain on physical grounds. They can, however, be found to have a relation with some sort of psychological stress. The patients have no conscious control over the symptoms.

They are not aware of the underlying cause.

In severe cases the symptoms can be paralysis blindness, deafness or hallucinations of different kinds. Very often there are vague symptoms like dizziness, loss of balance and co-ordination, headache, nausea, tics, tremors or numbness.

The conversion reaction is more common in females as compared to males. It is also common in young people.

Causes

The symptoms of conversion reaction are not imagined or malingered. They occur because there is some abnormality in the functioning of the brain. This can be proved by doing a functional

MRI of the brain. In case of a person who cannot move his limb, the f-MRI shows the signals in the brain being produced in the appropriate part of the cortex as would be seen in any normal person moving the limb. It shows that the patient intends to move the limb but the limb is still not moving, then the instruction of the brain is not being transmitted to the neighboring cortex which tells the muscles to move.

I Treat. He Cures– (Placebo Effect)

The human body has remarkable powers of recovery triggered by the mind to produce a wide range of healing effects. One way of activating this healing potential is to give the patient dummy treatment when the patient is not aware of the dummy aspect of it. The patient has faith in the doctor and his medicines. He thinks: "I will go to the family doctor. I have faith. The doctor will examine and give me medicine and I will be cured." This is self hypnosis. This in itself is the curative element; the medicine given is only a placebo. The patient feels the doctor has cured him. The doctor says, "I treat. He cures." Probably the most dramatic placebo of all can be surgery at times. It has been proved by randomized double blind clinical trials.

16 Diseases of The Mind

As has already been noted, no disease is purely physical but the human mind also plays some role in it. The following diseases show a greater role of the mind than the body. The first among them is Phobia.

Phobia means morbid fear. Phobia is an extreme form of anxiety and mental disorder. We know fear is a protective response in life. But when the fear is disproportionate to the cause, the sufferer tries to avoid confronting the cause.

The person is aware of the irrational excessive fear; still he cannot control it and shows an excessive pathological reaction or response to fear. If the sufferer cannot avoid it, he endures it with distress which interferes in his social and occupational activities. As the sufferer experiences the phobic stimulus, anxiety levels increase.

There are different types of Phobias, related to different objects: Animals like dogs, snakes, scorpions, cockroaches, lizards etc. It may be of a dark room, closed chambers, lift, flying, height, water, mirror, sexual organs or for many other things. There are specific names for different phobias.

Caligynophobia is fear of beautiful women, phallophobia is of the erect penis, catoprophobia of the mirror, cramophobia of money, clinophobia of sleep coitophobia of sex, epistimo phobia of knowledge, Pluto phobia of wealth, photophobia of lights, hydrophobia of water Odontophobia of dentists, acrophobia for heights, agoraphobia for open spaces and the worst narco phobia, of death. People may have phobias of public speaking, crowded areas or even of passing urine in public urinals.

Phobias vary in severity amongst individuals. Some individuals can simply avoid the subject of their fear and suffer relatively mild anxiety. Others suffer a full-fledged panic attack with disabling symptoms. The patients/victims, are aware that this fear response is out of proportion but cannot overcome their panic reaction. Phobias are classified among five subtypes: a) of animals, b) of natural environment, c) of blood, d)of injections e) of injury. f) of situations and others. The symptoms and signs of phobia include extreme panic attacks, breathlessness, palpitation, oppression, pain in the chest, tremors all over the body, giddiness, hot flushes, headaches, sweating, cold palms and feet, tingling, numbness, butter flies in the stomach, nausea, a feeling of going crazy, vomiting and so on. Sometimes there is a feeling of detachment from ones own body. Some people feel like running away from the scene. The sufferer is certainly aware that this is a disproportionate response to the stimulus but cannot overpower the fear.

Treatment

Phobias are chronic and tend to worsen if untreated. Fortunately, they can be treated successfully but the sufferer must have a desire to get rid of it. He has to co-operate with the psychiatrist for counseling and de-sensitization. Desensitization means showing pictures, videos of the objects producing the phobia. Somebody other than the doctor or relative can handle the objects causing the phobia without any harm. Yoga, pranayam and such other techniques of physical and mental relaxation can be practiced. If necessary, the physician can add a little anxiolytic medication. Most of the phobias can be overcome in this manner.

Phobia of all sorts like panic disorder and O.C.D. all fall in anxiety disorders.

"RIGHT and WRONG" (OCD)

Can we be right and wrong at the same time? Yes! It is possible. Cleanliness is right but if we are washing our hands every now and then it is wrong. If we are checking doors and windows to see if they are properly closed before going to bed, we are certainly right but if we are doing it seven or eight times and still not sure that we have checked them well, then we are wrong. It means our actions are going beyond reasonable precautions and still we are not being satisfied. It means we are obsessed by the thought of cleanliness or safety. We are doing it under compulsion again and again. It means the idea or thought is continually preoccupying our mind. These ideas are fixed in the mind. It becomes a passion, compulsion and addiction. We are going crazy.

When we see somebody obsessed with some such idea or act, it is called Obsessive Compulsive Disorder (O.C.D.). This is a type of anxiety disorder. The causes of anxiety can be Hypoxia of the brain due to some reason. It may be due to some hormonal imbalance or some inflammatory disease of the nervous system. Cognitive behavioral therapies as well as medicines can help in recovery.

O.C.D. takes a chronic course with waxing and waning of symptoms. It usually responds fairly to treatment, though at times it is resistant.

Schizo (Delusions)

The common man knows something about almost every common behavioral abnormality. It is not possible for him to know all the technical terms in medicine. Still he uses some of these terms, often loosely. Shall we attempt to educate him to a limited extent about some of the psychological ailments?

Schizophrenia is a fairly common mental disorder. The cause is unknown. There is a disturbance in the feeling, thinking and behavior of the person. Delusions and hallucinations are common. Speech and behavior is disorganized. They hear voices that do not go away. These people lack emotion and motivation. This usually starts in young adults but can develop at any age. Some of them remain mute, motionless and in bizarre postures, at times agitated without any apparent cause. The worst part is that they do not think they are abnormal. They resist treatment.

The near ones have to take a clue and take such persons to a psychiatrist. It is observed that those with positive symptoms respond well to medication than the ones with negative symptoms.

Combinations of genetic and environmental factors play a role in causing this disorder.

Psychiatrists treat it with medications, Electroconvulsive (ECT) shock therapy and counseling.

Anxiety

Fear is a proportionate response to a perceived actual threat. The person meets it with a fight or flight response which is in-built. This is the instinct that protects life.

Anxiety on the other hand is an excessive fear of an unknown or imaginary threat. Fear of imminent death is very common. Fear is a normal response but anxiety is an excessive response, disproportionate to the imagined threat. This leads to restlessness, fatigue, problems of concentration and muscular tension.

GAD

Generalized Anxiety Disorder is a mental disorder where a person has irrationally excessive worry about things in everyday life.

Subtypes of anxiety disorder include phobias – excessive fear of height, a closed compartment (elevator), water and many other things including sexual organs.

The physical symptoms seen are palpitations, increased heart rate, muscle weakness, tension, fatigue, nausea, chest pain, breathlessness and perspiration. There may be external signs of pallor, sweating, trembling and pupillary dilatation.

Thus anxiety could be defined as agony and terror disproportionate to the perceived or imagined threat. These patients/victims feel everything is scary.

Causes

Parental rejection, lack of parental warmth, harsh discipline, child abuse, drug abuse and sex-abuse are common causes. Some genetic factors like use of excessive caffeine are also a reason. Cognitive behavioral therapy and ECT are useful in such cases. In extreme cases psychosurgery is under trial.

Moods (Deprssion)

Every one wants to be in a good mood. However life is full of ups and downs. Moods do swing from pleasant euphoric to depressive.

Depression

In Depression, there is a loss of appetite but they may overeat as there is no satisfaction while eating. This may lead to obesity, mild or gross. These people cannot concentrate and memory and decision making is adversely affected. All this can lead to suicidal tendencies or suicide. They have aches, pains, insomnia or excessive sleep, fatigue and loss of energy.

Depression is a state of low mood and aversion to activity. It can affect a person's thought, behavior, feelings and sense of well-being. The person feels sad, anxious, empty, hopeless, worried, helpless, worthless, guilty, irritable and restless.

Depression is not necessarily a psychic disorder. It can be a normal reaction to depressing sad, or undesired events such as loss of a dear one, financial crises, loss of livelihood etc. There is short lived episodic depression in day to day life. The intensity goes down with time or with the solution of the problem. This can happen after childbirth, menopause and when diagnosed with diseases like HIV, cancers or after catastrophic injuries leading to loss of a limb.

Temporary depression may be due to certain medication. Drugs used for hepatitis C, betablockers or reserpine used for treatment of high blood pressure can cause depression.

Certain diseases like Addison's disease, multiple sclerosis, chronic pain, stroke, diabetes, cancer and sleep apnea and disturbance in sleep rhythm, hypothyroidism all can lead to depression.

Psychiatric Syndrome

The depressive mood disorder is a mood disorder which needs

attention and treatment from an expert psychiatrist. This is diagnosed if the person has at least two weeks of depressed mood.

These need antidepressant medicines, ECT and psychoanalytically oriented counselling.

Eating a healthy diet, exercise, meditation, stopping smoking along with a group and family therapy work well to address this.

Women are more prone to depression, possibly because of the gender role in the family. This disorder runs in families. Hormones also play a part.

Sexual Life

A happy married and social life leading to all round physical and mental satisfaction is a key factor in everybody's life. A proper sexual relationship is the most important factor for achieving such a satisfactory life though it may not be the only factor. To achieve this, the relationship should be satisfactory. This is important for both the partners. Both the sexual partners need to be physically and mentally prepared for the act. Everybody, whether educated, uneducated, blind, deaf or dumb is good at it. This is why we call it an instinct.

Sexual dysfunction

However, there are instances where the partners do not know what to do and how to perform. They need counseling. At times there are physical or physiological barriers. e.g, A tight or tough hymen in the female or an erectile dysfunction in the male.

Sexual dysfunction is defined as inability of the couple to have complete coitus or reach orgasm. Sexual dysfunction can be symptomatic (biological problems), interpersonal problems (or psychogenic) or a combination of both. This may be at the stage of desire, arousal or orgasm.

Causes

The causes in males can be physical or psychological. The psychological cause is often in the form of inadequate erection or early ejaculation. This can be due to anxiety, tension or depression. guilt, stress or physical fatigue, and lack of interest in the partner leading to lack of arousal. This was known earlier as impotence and now it is termed as erectile dysfunction.

This may also be due to physical causes reducing the blood flow to the penis. This includes diabetes, atherosclerosis due to aging or decreased levels of the hormone testosterone. Damage to the nerve erygentes during surgery of prostate or colorectal cancer also leads to erectile dysfunction. Certain diseases like syphilis and certain medicines especially antidepressants can cause erectile dysfunction. The problem of premature ejaculation can also be due to psychological or neurological causes. Nicotine, narcotics and stimulants also lead to erectile dysfunction in males.

Sildenaphil (Viagra) helps with erection if there are no other factors for the dysfunction. Alcohol is supposed to increase the desire but takes away the performance.

Causes in Females

Lack of sexual arousal in females is called frigidity. This may be psychological because of fear, dislike for the partner, due to anxiety, depression or physical aging, menopause, pregnancy, lactation or deficiency of hormones estrogen or testosterone.

There could be physical causes like tough intact hymen, lack of vaginal secretions required for lubrication or inflammation of genitalia leading to pain. Painful coitus in females is called dysparunia. Sometimes an ovary behind the uterus lower down can be the cause of the pain, sometimes the vaginal muscles go into spasm making the coitus painful and difficult.

A gentle attitude on the part of the male partner, enough foreplay, stimulation of the clitoris all go a long way in the arousal of the female which can help her have an orgasm. A hasty act may lead to ejaculation and orgasm to the male but may not help the female partner in reaching the climax. This may lead her to dissatisfaction.

A good ambience, tender music, scents and good time spent in foreplay and after-play can make the partners reach the climax and satisfy both.

In cases of physical problems a sex expert(sexologist) should be consulted. A psychiatrist can help if there is a psychological problem, especially if the lady has phallophobia (excess fear of the penis).

Defying Instinct - Suicidal Thought

Fear has been a life protecting instinct from times immemorial. Preserving life against all dangers or odds is a top priority of all life forms. Suicidal thinking (ideation) is not common. A person who is a victim of psychiatric disturbance is likely to be a victim of this thought.

Love, selflessness, altruism are prominent parts of human thinking. Altruism is easy to preach than practice. Our brain is prudent because it thinks of these high qualities or principles until they become a threat to life. Once a definite threat is perceived, the brain thinks otherwise. May I quote one of the stories of Akbar and Birbal to prove the point? Birbal asserted that life of one's own self has a priority even over that of the dearest offspring. He was asked to prove his point as the Emperor disagreed. Birbal kept the young one of a monkey and its mother in a dry well without an exit and started filling up the well with water. The mother monkey immediately lifted the baby and took it on her head to protect it. The Emperor thought that he had been proved right. As the water level started rising to the nose of the mother, she kept the baby down and stood on it to breathe for survival. Birbal was proved right.

If preserving ones own life from all sorts of dangers is the fundamental instinct of all life forms, why do some brains think of ending it? What is suicidal ideation?

Let it be clear first that such suicidal thoughts are exceptions and not a rule. A normal brain does not allow them. An extreme form of thinking disorders, with or without the physical and degenerative disorders of the brain, leads to this pathological thinking. Excessive anxiety or depression, very traumatizing experiences in life such as severe and unbearable pain with no hope of relief, loss of a loved one can also trigger such thoughts. The brain thinks that there is no chance of relief and no alternative left but to end life.

At times a disturbed person pretends to commit suicide to draw attention. Such a person plans only to fail and makes a cautious half-hearted attempt leaving some hints for others to act and save him. They usually try to see that they do not actually die. Very rarely is it a serious and successful attempt defying the instinct of self preservation and survival. Such people have a fixed plan to succeed. Signs and symptoms exhibited by the patients vary. They look moody, anxious, exhibit change of personality, change of routine, change in sleeping patterns etc. They consume drugs or alcohol, drive carelessly, try to get hold of a gun or a knife. They may show signs of depression or panic disorder.they often tend to criticize themselves, remain isolated, say good bye to others as if for the last time and keep away from pleasurable social events, exercise and sex. These people talk about killing themselves and express regret for being alive or born.

Psychiatric Emergencies

Those who are serious about their plan to commit suicide often create emergency situations by a serious attempt on their own self or become violent and can harm others including the doctor.

Men commit suicide more commonly than women. People above 40-50 are more prone to commit suicide.

Addiction – An Invited Curse

We considered the defying instinct of suicide in the last page. People use various substances for having a pleasant sensation. Nobody starts taking alcohol or drugs with an intention of becoming an addict. The pleasure sensation varies from a feeling of light headedness, a sense of floating or flying, a sense of nirvana to euphoria. Once experienced, the person wants to re-experience it again and again. The desire for pleasure is inbuilt in the brain. Gradually the quantity of the substance needs to be increased for having the same effect. This is known as tolerance to the substance. Next, there is a physiological (physical) or psychological dependence of the person on the substance to function normally. Once this stage is reached the person craves for the substance. He will try his best to get it by all means, fair and foul, despite the knowledge about adverse effects of the substance on physical and mental health. If deprived of the substance, the person shows different signs and symptoms grouped together as withdrawal symptoms.

> Addiction is a curse because it is suicidal. It starts with a pleasant sensation but the end is dire.

There are various withdrawal symptoms are various like craving for the substance, having nausea, vomiting, diarrhea, muscle ache, headache, watering of the eyes and nose, pupillary dilatation, sweating, fever, loss of sleep, difficulty in swallowing, fatigue, agitation, anxiety, increased sensitivity to light and sound, coarse tremors and epileptic fits.

Treatment

Prevention is the best policy. The people who have seen addicts in the family or around must avoid all such addictive substances. Not to smoke or drink is in no way anti-social. False ideas of socializing must be done away with. It has to be understood that these substances are not the remedy for anxiety, tension or fatigue. In fact, they are the means of inviting them all and much more.

However, if your dear ones are victims, it is your prime duty to take them to a psychiatrist or to an anonymous center where group therapies are being carried out. Once addicted to drugs, nothing short of it is likely to succeed. It is likely to be a long drawn, systematic battle.

It would be worthwhile going through a list of addicting substances we should be aware of.

Alcohol, tobacco, amphetamines, caffeine, cannabis, cocaine, opiates, heroin, sedative and anxiolytic medicines, LSD and many more addictive substances are in use by many addicts all around us. This list is not exhaustive.

Mechanism of action

Dopamine is the primary neurotransmitter of the reward (pleasure) system in the brain. These recreational substances cause a release of dopamine. Nearly all addictive drugs, directly or indirectly, act upon the brain's reward system by heightening dopamine activity. The brain gains short term pleasure but is misled into a trap of long lasting disasters. BEWARE OF THEM!

Pleasure

Pleasure is preferred to food and water. Dopamine and sexotonin connect the various pleasure centers in the brain The dopamine rush is linked to the experienced after taking drugs.

Aliens Controlling Brain

In schizophrenic patients the mechanism that monitors intentions and compares it with performance is flawed, a more bizarre interpretation is likely to result , such as the body movements are controlled by aliens or brain implants, which is what paranoid schizophrenics claim

Dead Person is Alive (cotard's syndrome)

Is it a correct statement? Possibly not but in Cotards Syndrome the patient really claims he or she is dead. In these patients the vision other the senses are disconnected from the emotional centers. So that nothing in the world has any emotional significance, the only way in which a patient can interpret this complete emotional desolation is to believe that he or she is dead. Once this delusional fixation develops, all contrary evidence is warped to accommodate it.

Mini Cotard Syndrome

This is more commonly seen than Cotard's syndrome. This Mini Cotard's is known as derealisation and depolarization, and is found in acute anxiety, panic attacks, depression and other dissociative state.

James Bond

If a lion attacks a man and mauls an arm, a soldier loses a limb in war, or a woman is being raped or such dire emergencies, the anterior cingulate gyrus in the brain, becomes extremely active. This inhibits or temporarily shuts down the amygdala and other limbic emotional centers, so temporarily suppressing potentially disabling emotions such as anxiety and fear. But at the same time the anterior cingulate activation generates extreme alertness and vigilance in preparation for any appropriate defensive reaction that might be required.

In an emergency, this is the James Bond like combinations of shutting down emotions (nerve of steel) while being hypervigilant for fight or flight.

But what if the same mechanism is accidentally triggered by chemical imbalance or brain diseases, when there is no emergency? The patient takes fight or flight and fright for no reason. For him ' the world is not real' this is derealisation or , he feels ' I am not real'- this is depersonasation .

(MENTAL ILLNESS) Evolutionary Neuro psychiatry

Try to identify chemical imbalances, changes in neurotransmitters and receptors in the brain and attempt to correct these changes using medicines.

Multiple Personality Disorder

Even people with so called multiple personality disorders don't experience two personalities simultaneously. The personalities tend to rotate and are mutually amnesic.

NEURO CRIMINOLOGY

A time may come when we may be able to do brain scans to

determine whether a defendant is guilty of premeditated murder or merely of manslaughter.

17 Symptoms of Brain Diseases

Pain Friend!

Pen friends are those created with a pen. Also, the pen is our best friend. But we never consider pain as our friend. We try to avoid it in any condition. Doctors give their patients medicines or injections as pain killers because we feel pain is our foe. But actually pain is not our foe, it is our friend. This is the bitter truth. Bitter medicine is a friend because it is useful for health; similarly pain is also useful for health. Pain is indeed our friend. It makes us aware of injurious stimuli and tells us to draw ourselves away from such objects or things which damage our body. So a friend in need is a friend indeed. This applies to pain mechanism as well.

Pain is one of our most useful survival mechanisms. What we feel as pain, however, does not necessarily match up with what is happening to our body because pain is like everything we experience.'It is all in the mind.'

If we take the example of a painful stimulus, the severity of pain felt is inversely proportional to the amount of attention we can pay at that moment. Suppose, we are conscious and a needle pricks us or something stings our body, we take our hand away with lightning speed. But if we are engrossed in some important task of our interest and are not attentive, even a bigger painful stimulus may not hurt us or will hurt very less. Unless we pay attention to the information coming in from the senses, we are not conscious of it.

Neurophysiology of Pain

On the other hand, we may experience pain in the absence of pain signals coming from outside. It all depends on the mind. This is known as the neuropathic pain, but this pain is not imaginary, it is a form of memory. We continue to feel pain even after an injury has healed. This is because of the wiring together of brain cells even after healing. This neuropathic pain is seen in certain diseases of the nerves like diabetes.

> Pain signals from the nerves in the skin, muscles and joints enter the somato-sensory cortex of the brain. This does not automatically produce a painful experience. Another part of the brain has to bring the signals to consciousness by directing attention to them. When this process is complete, we feel pain.

Congenital Insensitivity to Pain - Pain Asymbolia

Pain alerts us to beware of injury. It is a useful warning system. Painlessness is rarely an abnormality found in a newborn child. The exact mechanism of this defect has not yet been understood. James was one such child. He had no pain sensation. This child was very much injury-prone and often used to sustain burns, cuts and fractures. His mother Ruth had to fight a constant battle to keep him out of danger. James was otherwise a bright and sensible child but doctors could not help the child. Such children have a shorter than normal life span. Genetic research is on to understand the mechanism.

PAIN ASYMBOLIA

Vilaynur Ramachadran reported such a case. The patient responded to pain stimulus not with an 'ouch' but with laughter. Laughter is nature's OK signal. CT scan of the brain of the patient showed damage to the insular cortex. The insular cortex receives pain signals from the viscera and from the skin. From the insular cortex, the message goes to the amygdala , and then to the rest of the limbic system and especially the anterior cingulategyrus, where we respond emotionally to the pain. So perhaps in this patient the insular cortex was normal, so he could feel the pain, but the wire that goes from the insula to the rest of the limbic system and the anterior cingulate was cut. Such a situation would produce the two key ingredients required for laughter and humour : If this connection between insula and the limbic system is deficient at birth, it is dubbed as congenital pain asymbolia.

This is why I say that pain is a friend. A real friend!

Let us be-friend pain. Pain is an unpleasant feeling caused by damaging stimuli such as pricking, cutting, burning etc. Pain is a disagreeable sensory and emotional experience associated with actual or potential tissue damage. Yet, it is a fact that it alerts us to withdraw from damaging situations, protects the damaged part till it heals, and helps us avoid such damaging situations in future.

Pain is a major symptom in many medical conditions. Pain is said to be acute or severe when it is of a sudden onset and lasts for a few months (1 to 6 months). The pain lasting for longer time is termed as chronic. Pain can be localized, or spread over an area. It may be continuous, dull aching or intermittent colicky (spasmodic). It may be mild, moderate or severe. It may be at the site of the injury or may be referred to some other area supplied by the same segmental nerve. Common examples are tongue or throat pain referred to the ear or ureteric pain referred to the testicle.

GOOD NEIGHBORS (PHANTOMS IN BRAIN)

Sensations of pain in a limb amputated due to disease or after injury is called phantom sensation. The phantom is in the brain. The cause is a good neighbor act.

Dr. Vilayanur Ramchandran reported such a case. The person's left arm was amputated above the elbow and he was blindfolded during the testing. Different areas of his body were touched. When his left cheek was touched he exclaimed 'Oh my god, you are touching my left thumb'. When his upper lip was touched, he thought it was his missing index finger, the lower jaw, he believed to be his phantom little finger. There was a complete, systematic map of the missing phantom hand draped on his face.

This is a good neighborly act by the adjacent area in the brain. Representation of the face on the brain map is right next to the representation of the hand. When an arm is amputated, no signals are received by the part of the brain's cortex corresponding to the hand. It becomes hungry for sensory input and the sensory input from the facial skin now invades the adjacent vacant territory which corresponds to the missing hand.

Psychalgia is a psychogenic pain. This is caused by prolonged mental, emotional or behavioral factors. The commonest in this category are headaches. People tend to feel that it is not real. However scientists feel that it is no less real than the pain from other sources.

This 'remapping' or 'cross wiring' is confirmed by brain imagining technique called magneto encephalagraphy (MEG).

Phantom Pain

The patients who have undergone an amputation of the limb sometimes complain of pain in the part which has been removed (amputated long back.) Such sensation of pain from the lost part of the body is phantom pain. These patients are not malingering. The cut portion of the nerve coming from the amputated part actually sends signals to the brain (due to some irritation at the cut end) and the brain interprets it as coming from the part that is no more in existence. At times such phantom pain can be removed with injection of a local anesthetic into the nerve.

Many times pain is labeled as psychogenic when the cause cannot be detected by the physician. This can be a folly. This could be our ignorance as of today and our inability to find out the cause.

Pain Thresholds

Different races in different geographies exhibit different thresholds for heat, electrical shock and other pain stimuli. Individuals in the same race also have wide variations. The pain perception threshold is the point at which the stimulus begins to hurt and the pain tolerance threshold is reached when the subject acts to stop the pain. f-MRI brain scanning is useful to measure pain, giving good correlations with self reported pain.

Headache for Doctors

To find out the exact cause of a headache in a patient and treat it successfully is often a headache for the physician as well. Headache is pain anywhere in the region of the head or the neck. It is a symptom of many conditions. The periosteum (nutritive covering of bones), muscles, nerves, arteries, veins, tissue below the skin, teeth, eyes, ears, sinuses and the inner lining of mouth (mucosa), any one of them can be the culprit. Treatment of headaches should be directed to the elimination of the cause but often failure to find out the exact cause necessitates symptomatic treatment with pain killer medicines or local application of counter irritants.

There are more than 200 causes for headache. Some may be harmless while others may be life threatening. 90% of primary headaches have no known cause; they are not life threatening; whether they are mild or severe like migraine. The secondary headache is a symptom of some primary disease, often a dangerous one, like meningitis, encephalitis (infections of brain or meninges) or brain tumors. 90% of headaches belonging to the primary category start in adolescence (20-40 yrs). The most common among these are due to common cold (nose being blocked), migraine and tension headache. Cough, sneezing, exercise and strain can increase primary headache. So also sex, orgasm and even sleep can induce primary headaches in some individuals. Tension headaches are thought to be caused by activation of peripheral nerves in the head and neck.

Migraine

Migraine is a long standing (chronic) neurological disorder. The headache caused is recurrent and from moderate to severe. It is often associated with watering of the eyes and nose (autonomic nervous system symptoms). Typically, the headache is one sided, (one side of the head pains) lasting from 2-72 hours. It may be associated with nausea, vomiting and sensitivity to light, sound or smell. The pain gets worsened with physical exercise. About a third of the sufferers get a warning aura - a transient, visual and sensory language or a motor disturbance before the onset of migraine.

Causes –

The causes are not precisely known. It is thought to be a genetic or an environmental factor. In about two third of the cases it runs in the family like a family business! Changing hormone levels like puberty, menarche and menopause bring in migraine, while pregnancy halts it. Migraine is more common in males before puberty and in females around and after puberty.

The exact mechanisms of headaches with migraine are not known. Formerly it was thought to be vascular in origin but now the focus is on neurovascular causes. It is thought to be due to the increased excitability of the cerebral cortex and abnormal control of pain neurons in the trigeminal nucleus of the brainstem.

Migraine has three phases: prodrome (foreplay phase), the aura, (pain phase) and the following or postdrome (after play phase).

Triggers

Stress, hunger, fatigue, menstruation, oral contraception, pregnancy, menopause all seem to trigger migraine. Blood examination indicates high levels of the neurotransmitter, serotonin.

Diagnosis

Two attacks with aura, five attacks without aura, unilateral headache, pulsating, moderate to severe pain, aggravation due to physical activity, nausea or vomiting, sensitivity to light and sound all go in favor of migraine. Prevention includes medications, nutritional supplements, alteration in lifestyle and at times surgery.

Medication, surgery should all be with consultation of the specialists. The outcome or recovery is variable. The symptoms can become less severe with time, may continue at the same frequency and severity or increase. Lucky are those whose migraine gets completely cured.

Trigeminal Neuralgia (TN)

This is a neuropathic disorder with moments of intense pain in the face originating from the trigeminal nerve. This is the most painful condition known to human beings. It is commonly seen after the age of 50 years, but no age is a bar and it is more common in the fair sex. The incidence of TN is increasing.

The trigeminal nerve is the V paired cranial nerve having three major divisions supplying the regions of the eye maxilla and the mandible (lower jaw). One two or all of the three regions on one or both sides may be involved. The pain type is severe, cutting, stabbing, electric shock, pressing, crushing, shooting and burning or exploding types. Pain may be felt in the ear, eye, lips, nose, scalp, forehead, teeth or jaws and side of the face. Life becomes hell. The pain is so severe that it leads to suicidal thoughts.

This pain is not controlled easily and is very incapacitating. It can last from seconds, minutes to hours. This pain can be easily triggered by touch, or an air current, high pitched sounds, loud noises, chewing, talking and brushing teeth. Recent studies indicate that it may be the compressing or throbbing against the micro vessels of the trigeminal nerve near its connection with the pons that cause pain. Such compression can injure the protective (myelin) sheath of the nerve, leading to erratic and hyperactive functioning of the nerve. Brain imaging technique like C.T. & MRI are of no avail

Fainting is a common and dramatic event witnessed by us in day to day life. You may be a spectator or the main actor in this drama.

Treatment

Proper evaluation by a specialist is mandatory. Easy diagnosis and prompt, proper treatment can reverse the problem. Delay must be avoided to hasten chances of recovery otherwise they become remote.

Good medication is available. It becomes difficult to go out independently if you are taking medicines If medical treatment fails, surgery may be contemplated with calculated chances of recovery. Procedures such as Radio Frequency Lesioning (RFL) or injections of glucol or alcohol - all are for numbing the nerve. These are Destructive ,methods. The other option is micro-Vascular Decompression which separates the blood vessel from the trigeminal nerve to take away pressure which is the cause of the problem. A sponge is interposed between the nerve and the blood vessel by surgery.

"Dramatic Fainting" - Vasovagal Syncope

The most common cause of fainting is a vasovagal syncope. It is mediated through the vagus nerve and acts through reduction of blood pressure and heart rate. Reduced heart rate and blood pressure reduce the output of the heart leading to reduction of oxygen and glucose vital for the functioning of the all important brain. This leads to fainting. If the person is sitting or standing at the moment of fainting, he is likely to collapse or fall down like a log of wood. Fainting usually vanishes(ends) in a second or a minute. It may not leave any trace of the event except an injury if the person falls down. This vasovagal syncope is common in young adults.

Signs and Symptoms

Generally there is some triggering factor. The individual may experience lightheadedness, nausea, a feeling of being extremely hot or cold. There may be an uncomfortable feeling in the heart, fuzzy thoughts, confusion and some difficulty in speech, weakness and visual disturbances and nervousness. If the person has become horizontal after fainting, the blood supply to the brain is improved and there is an equally dramatic recovery. The person becomes conscious. If the person is not horizontal, the oxygen deprivation to the brain can lead to a seizure (fit). The bye standers must make the person horizontal and turn the neck up and to one side. He should be left horizontal for sometime even after recovering consciousness. This prevents recurrence of the fainting.

The affected person becomes pale, there is cold sweating all over the body, the pulse rate is reduced and blood pressure becomes low.

Causes

Vasovagal syncope is triggered by many factors. A prolonged standing or sitting position and standing up suddenly after getting up from the bed especially if medicines for lowering blood pressure are being taken, can cause fainting. Extreme stress due to any reason, especially very severe pain of any origin can be another cause. Trivial triggers such as: sight of blood, surgery, sudden extreme emotions, even stimulants such as sex can cause fainting. Lack of sleep, dehydration and severe hunger, exposure to very high temperature, alcohol, cocaine, marijuana and inhaled opiates can all be triggering factors. Markedly reduced blood sugar is often seen in diabetics under treatment.

The vasovagal fainting is in short a cardio-inhibitory response to one of the above factors. Avoidance of these triggers prevents vasovagal syncope.

Spinning - Vertigo

A feeling of rotating or spinning is a common symptom of vertigo. A common cause is being paroxysmal positional. It comes at repeated intervals, only on changing the position of the head and neck. Though the patient feels frightened, it is harmless. It is related to the disorder of the inner ear.

Symptoms-

The spinning dizziness lasts with the rotational component from seconds to minutes only. Nausea is often present but vomiting is rare. There may be difficulty in seeing and reading because of the nystagmus (side to side or rotational involuntary movements of eye). Fainting or syncope in such attacks is unusual.

Menieres Disease

This is a disorder of the inner ear. The person has vertigo which is rotational or spinning in nature. It is unpredictable, severe and incapacitating. It lasts from minutes to hours but usually for less than 24 hour sand very rarely for weeks. There is a ringing noise in the ear and temporary but significant hearing loss. The hearing improves when the attack ends but gets worse and permanent with repeated attacks. The hearing loss is unilateral and fluctuating but gets bilateral and permanent with progress of the pressure or fullness in one or both ears. Nausea, vomiting, sweating and falling down occur when the disease progresses.

Vestibular Neuronitis

This is again, a problem of the inner ear nerve (Vestibular nerve). It may surface as a single episode or may manifest at intervals, leading to vertigo. This happens generally on one side. There may be associated nausea, vomiting & previous common cold.

Signs and symptoms

Mainly vertigo which occurs suddenly may lead to nausea and vomiting. It does not lead to hearing loss like Menieres disease. At times there are abnormal eye movements (Nystagmus).

Cerebellar Stroke Syndrome

This condition results when blood supply to the small brain (cerebellum) is drastically compromised due to any reason.

Signs and symptoms are vertigo, headache, vomiting and loss of balance (ataxia). This condition should not be mistaken for other conditions causing vertigo, nausea and vomiting. There is no spinning;(but) there is a definite loss of balance in this condition. A C.T. scan will show an infarct of the cerebellum. This condition needs to be treated promptly, otherwise it may prove fatal.

Spondylosis

Spondylosis is a common term and what it means is pain in the neck or the lumber region. Let us know a little more about this common malady. Spondylosis is a pain in the region of the neck. It makes the neck stiff and at times pain is referred to the shoulder and upper limb. In addition to pain, there may be tingling, numbness in the arm, forearm and hands. In severe cases there may be wasting of the muscles leading to muscle weakness. When this is restricted to the vertebrae of the neck, it is called cervical Spondylosis. If the pain, tingling or numbness is in the back or lower limb with or without muscle wasting, it is called Lumbar Spondylosis. Thus there may be sensory and motor symptoms depending on the nerve being compressed or irritated.

This can occur at any age but it is more common with the degenerative changes of advanced age. The degenerative changes in the intervertebral disc (prolapsed disc) can press the spinal cord or the nerve roots. There may be a pressure on the nerve roots either through the protruding discs or through the osteophytes (beak like projections) from the vertebral bodies, the bony arch or from the facet joints in between the vertebrae; or there may be a narrowing of the canal through which the spinal cord is passing down

Sciatica

Sciatica is another term familiar to the common man. When the sciatic nerve (the major nerve supplying the lower limb) is being compressed, there is severe pain radiating from the hip region down to the entire leg or part of the leg. There may be tingling, numbness and muscle wasting in addition. This neuralgic pain because of the compression of the sciatic nerve is called sciatica. If the disc is pressing on the lumbo-sacral nerves, there may be a disturbance in the bladder and bowel control.

> It is said that yawning occurs more when the atmospheric pressure drops after sunset and hence many people yawn at the same time. Yawning is useful to alert the brain.

C.T. and M.R.I scans after a thorough orthopaedic and neurological examination can give almost pinpoint diagnosis and level of compression.

Treatment

It is conservative at first. Modification of lifestyle, non-steroidal anti-inflammatory drugs and physiotherapy are a part of the treatment. If the symptoms do not wane and if there is anesthesia or muscle wasting, then surgery for decompression is required.

In olden days it used to be a mutilating surgery with morbidity. Now, the surgery can be performed with smaller incisions using windows for removal of the compressing disc or with a minimally invasive technique (like endoscopy). With these modern techniques the morbidity and loss of working hours is markedly reduced.

Yawning

Yawning is not the sole prerogative of human beings. Animals also yawn. It is seen in the young and old alike. Researchers have not been able to pin point the cause as yet. A common experience is that it happens when a person is tired, bored or feeling sleepy. The most common theory says it is the process by which the brain demands more oxygen and wants to reduce the carbon dioxide level in the blood. This is achieved by reflex stimulation leading to simultaneous deep inhalation with jaws widely opened and stretching of the ear drums followed by exhaltation of breath. It is a common observation that yawning appears to be contagious.

This is understandable because it leads to deep inhalation. It is also funny to note that even if you see, hear and read about yawning, it induces yawning. So it is thought that the yawning may be physiological as well as psychological. Thus it seems to be contagious, but the reasons behind it are unclear.

Yawning has been reported by a researcher in an eleven week foetus. But, we know for sure that the lungs do not open up and function till birth. We also know for sure that deep inhalation is the beginning of the process and an integral part of yawning. Hence, it is not possible for a foetus to yawn.

In yawning the mouth opens, the jaw drops allowing as much air as possible to be taken in. The lungs expand to capacity and then you blow back some air yawning leads to the opening of the pulmonary alveoli which may have closed during a prolonged period of quiet breathing. The deep (inhalation) also increases the venous return to the heart leading to increased cardiac output.

This is a person's natural defence against a buildup of carbon dioxide in the blood. Whenever oxygen levels in the blood drop, the brain will order yawning. The stretching of arms commonly associated with yawning strangely causes movement of even paralysed limbs which cannot be voluntarily moved. This is difficult to explain but is true. This is called pandiculation which is also a reflex action.

Some researchers have concluded that the viruses of the common cold use host manipulation to their advantage. They induce sneezing and are thrown in the air in the form of droplets.

Excessive yawning is found in some pathological conditions such as sleep disorders (sleep apnea), medications used for anxiety and depression, vasoragal reactions, and heart attacks. At times, it is associated with epilepsy following encephalitis, brain stroke, brain tumor, liver failure and in opiate addicts.

Sneezing

Can we stop a sneeze? Probably not. Sneezing is a reflex induced by the brain to guard against the foreign particles from the respiratory passage to the lungs and the body. The medical term for sneezing is sternutation. It is a complex co-ordinated action between the brain, nerves and muscles all over the body.

Our nose is lined with microhair called cilia. They catch foreign particles such as pollens, dander and microbes. When these tickle the inner lining of the nose, the brain receives a message to send the particles out. The brain orders abdominal muscles and chest muscles to contract which initiates a forceful current of air out through the wind pipe, throat and nasal passages.

The common factors leading to sneezing are smoke, pollution, moulds, dust, pollens, strong fumes or odour. Animal dander, allergens, cold air and even bright sunlight can trigger cases of photic sneeze. The last one has a genetic basis.

The viruses in those droplets get an easy access to another host, thus serving their purpose of survival and propagation. We dance to the tune of this guest.

Laughter the best Medicine

Laughter is provoked or produced by pleasant sensation. Be they tickling or jokes Laughter acts mainly through the hypothalamus us, through the left and right brain the frontal lobe, and the sensory motor cortex of the brain. All are involved in the process. All these actions are mediated by the neurotramsmitter dopamine. This improves immunity which improves health.

Hiccup

Hiccups are a common day-to-day experience irrespective of age. Most often they are short lived and do not warrant any attention or treatment. There is actually no definite cause. The typical sound and sensation during a hiccup is produced by the diaphragm; the muscle that separates chest and abdomen, when it contracts with a sudden jerk. The contraction forces us to take a quick breath. It is annoying but seldom painful.

These spasms are caused by irritation of the phrenic nerve, the nerve of the diaphragm. The sound is produced by the closure of the oesophagus by the epiglottis as the breath is rushing in.

Causes

Some reasons for this are eating or drinking quickly, stress or nervousness, alcohol, spicy foods, crying or laughing hard etc. but most of the times it is without an apparent cause. Other causes are the reflux of stomach acid in the oesophagus and irritation of the throat. Chronic hiccups lasting for hours or days or weeks are attributed to medications, metabolic disorders (uremia) and neurological damage to the brainstem.

Treatment

No particular treatment is known to be effective. The drugs used are baclofen, chlorpromazine, metclopromide, gabapentin and proton pump inhibitors.

If there is a disease responsible for the hiccups it can be treated. The phrenic nerve can be blocked temporarily with 0.5% procaine or permanently with bilateral phrenicotomy. Nothing however, can guarantee a cure. If it is due to electrolyte imbalance, it can be corrected. Implanting the vagus nerve stimulating device may help.

Making Faces and Crocodile Tears

We often see people making faces. It is a deliberate act. But sometimes making faces may not be a voluntary and deliberate act but the result of the paresis or paralysis of the facial nerve. If tears are shed without any sorrow, they are called Crocodile Tears .They are a hypocritical show of sorrow. Persons suffering from facial palsy shed tears while chewing food without sorrow or unpleasant feelings. We can call them crocodile tears in a lighter vein.

Actually, the facial nerve mainly controls the muscles of the forehead, the eyelids, the lachrymal (tear) apparatus and muscles around the mouth and the secretions of the salivary gland. The effect on the face is generally on one side but rarely it can be on both sides. Besides the weakness of the facial muscles, there may be increased hearing or decreased tears and saliva on the affected side. There may also be loss of taste on the affected side. Facial palsy is common in diabetic patients.

The infection of herpes zoster, the middle ear, the fracture of the ear bone (temporal), a tumor of the brain, an infarct of the brain in the region of the internal capsule, pons or in neighboring area can produce facial nerve palsy. C.T. or MRI of the brain are useful tools after taking the history and doing neurological examination. Bell's Palsy is diagnosed after exclusion of all the above causative factors. It is because of the dysfunction of the facial nerve. 80% of the facial palsies fall under the category of Bell's Palsy.

The person having facial palsy due to any cause is unable to close the eye on the affected side. He cannot blink it. The affected side of the face shows weakness or paralysis of muscles while smiling, frowning, flaring nostrils and raising eyebrow. Lacrimation and salivation on the affected side are reduced but movement of the eyelids is lost and hence tears come down the cheeks involuntarily.

All this happens due to inflammation of the facial nerve which comes out through a rigid bony canal. Bell's Palsy patients can recover within 3 weeks. Steroids help in early recovery. If recovery does not occur in 3 weeks the physician must look for and treat the primary cause. In that case it is not Bell's palsy.

If it is an irreversible paralysis of the facial nerve, surgery is advised to make the eyelids close; otherwise corneal ulceration can lead to blindness. Similarly, the angle of the mouth draws to one side while laughing speaking, and eating. But, it can be corrected by plastic surgery procedures.

PARALYSIS OF LIMBS

Paralysis of one or more limbs can occur. If one limb is involved it is called monoplegia. If two limbs are involved, it is paraplegia and if all the four are involved, it is called quadruplegia.

Congenital causes like cerebral palsy and spina bifida can cause paralysis of one or two limbs. Infections like tuberculosis of the spine and traumatic injuries to the spine involving the spinal cord or a nerve is a common cause of paralysis of limbs. The lower limbs are affected if there is injury to thoracic or lumber vertebra but all the four limbs will be affected in infections and injuries to the vertebra of the neck. If the injury is at the 4th cervical vertebra or above, it can lead to respiratory paralysis because the nerves to the diaphragm (the main muscle of respiration) are paralyzed. These patients are prone to pressure sores (bed sores), thrombosis in veins and pneumonias.

In cases of paraplegia (both legs) and quadruplegia (all four limbs), besides paralysis of muscles, control of urine and bowel is also lost. Much care is required to avoid pressure sores, and extensive physiotherapy is needed for bladder and bowel care. Use of stem cells for regeneration of damaged spinal cord is still in the experimental stage.

Beware of Unethical Propaganda And Malpractices In This Respect.

Terrible Excitement - Epilepsy

Whenever some unexpected and pleasant surprise comes our way, we get excited. We enjoy and share our excitement with others. However, our brain does not like an unexpected and unusual excitement of any of its parts. If it occurs in any part of the cerebral cortex, it can be recorded in a graphic manner. We call it Electro Encephalograms (EEG). Such unexpected, unusual excitement of cerebral cortex leads to epileptic seizure. The commonest type of epilepsy is called grandmal epilepsy.

Grandmal Epilepsy

In this type of epilepsy, the person may have some premonitory symptoms (aura) like nonexistent smells, noises in the ears, or flashes of light. Then tonic convulsions begin in one part of the body and may involve the entire body. There is frothing from the mouth. There may be tongue bite, that is, the person may bite his or her own tongue, lose consciousness and falls down. There may be vomiting or involuntary evacuation of the bowels or bladder. These seizures vary from very brief and almost undetectable duration to long periods of vigorous shaking of a part of or the complete body. They tend to recur. and become a chronic problem. The seizures can be controlled in about 70% of the cases but cannot be completely cured. About 1% of the population suffers from epilepsy.

The epileptic seizures occur more often during sleep. The person may make a loud noise because of contraction of the muscles of the chest. After regaining consciousness and following a seizure, the person may have headache, tiredness, difficulty in speaking and an abnormal behavior. Some of these people develop depression, anxiety and migraines. Genetic defect in one or more genes is thought to be responsible and hence, we see many members in the family suffering from epileptic seizures. Epilepsy has no known cause.

Secondary Seizures

Infection of the central nervous system, brain damage following trauma (scarring), difficult childbirth (Forceps delivery), brain tumors, cerebral cavernous and arterio venous malformations, and meningitis are some factors that can lead to epilepsy. Tapeworm infestations (neurocysticercosis), cerebral malaria and many other diseases can produce convulsive seizures. They are the symptoms of some other disease. Every effort must be made to find and treat the primary cause. EEG, C.T. and MRI scans after thorough history and clinical examinations are useful. CSF examination after lumbar puncture is often useful.

Diagnosis of Epilepsy

Diagnosis of Epilepsy is essentially one of exclusion of other diseases but an EEG can be useful.

Treatment –

The person should be turned to one side during seizures. A tongue depressor or an airway is inserted in the mouth to avoid obstruction to the airway. In case the attacks are continuous it is called status epilepticus. These patients need to be cared for in the ICU. The neurophysician uses phenobarbitone, diazepam and phenytoin for medication. If there are no seizures for 2-4 years then medication can be stopped only to restart if needed.

Evolutionery nero psychiatry

Try to identify chemical imbalances ,changes in nero transmitters and receptors in the brain and attempt to correct these changes using medicines

Synesthesia (Hear The Colours)

The cross-wiring in the brain that results mostly from amputation can also occur owing to a gene mutation. This accidental cross-wiring results in a curious condition called synesthesia. (First documented by Francis Galton in the nineteenth century.) In such patients hearing a particular musical note might invoke a particular colour : C sharp is red, F sharp is blue etc.

Fusiform gyrus is the area of the brain that houses both visual graphemes of numbers and colour information almost touching each other. Synesthesia is more common among people who use LSD.

Face Blindnees (Prosopognosia)

Vision is a very complex process. It involves the eyes optic nerve & about thirty different areas of the cerebral cortex which analyse the information received from the eyes in order for you to identify the object seen. This identification is partly done in a small area called fusifdm gyrus . If there is damage to this part, it leads to face blindness or prosopognosia. The patient can see, read books but cannot identify faces of people.

Capgras Syndrome

When after an accidental trauma to the brain, the patient recognizes the faces of dear ones but feels that they are imposters, it is called Capgras Syndrome. This happens if the wires in the brain joining the visual and emotional centers are cut. However he can still recognize the voice of the dear one on phone.

Colour Blind & Motion Blind

Thirty areas in visual cortex are specialized in different aspects of vision. One area called V4 is concerned only with colour information, for the most part. Another area named MT, or the middle temporal area, is concerned mainly with seeing motion. If V4 is damaged on both sides of the brain the result is colour blindness. If the MT, is damaged, a patient cannot tell the direction in which something is moving, or how fast it is moving. Such patients are scared of walking on or crossing the streets.

Neglect Syndrome

The parietal lobes are concerned with creating a symbolic representation of the spatial layout of the external world. The ability of spatial navigation: avoiding obstructions, dodging a flying object, catching a ball. Damage to the right parietal lobe produces the neglect syndrome. The patient no more moves his eyes towards the object which is looming towards him from the left. The person becomes indifferent to the left side & vice versa.

18 Diseases of The Nervous System

Parkinson's Disease-

Degenerative diseases in general, and those of the brain in particular are a flipside of the longevity given to human race by the advancement in medical science and technology through medicine and surgery. Parkinson's is a complex symptom seen in certain diseases. Parkinson's disease (P.D.) and Alzheimer's disease are the prominent degenerative disorders of the brain. Except degenerative changes no other causative factors are known as of today. The dopamine levels in the brain are reduced. There is degeneration of substantianigra, a small part of the brain and in the dopaminergic neural tracts. It is observed more commonly in people after repeated trauma to the head and also in those who use synthetic heroin. Parkinsons Disease is a movement disorder during later years of life. It is characterized by slow movements, resting tremors, pill rolling tremors and a mask-like face, cogwheel rigidity and a shuffling gait. Intellectual impairment and depression are common. This disease is found in 0.002% of population. Majority of the patients have dementia.

Treatment

There is no known preventive or curative treatment. Dopamine precursor drugs,Larodopa and Carbidopa are used for increasing dopamine levels in the brain. Some surgeons have tried implanting Adrenal medulla tissue into the brain to produce Dopamine with some favorable results. Depression associated with P.D. can be treated with antidepressants or E.C.T. Non-medicinal treatment may be useful to a limited extent. It includes physical and occupational therapy. These are all symptomatic treatments. Treating the disease relieves the symptoms.

Psychosomatic Disorders

The parts of the brain like hypothalamus, pituitary and the adrenal gland lead to an increase in stress hormones(cortisol) in response to mental stress. This reduces the immunity of the body and causes structural damage to various organ systems. This makes the body more vulnerable to infection, cancer and other disorders.

Psychosomatic disorders by definition are those physical illnesses in which mental factors play a significant role in the development, expression or resolution of the illness. Persons who are chronically anxious or depressed are more vulnerable to physical or psychosomatic diseases.

Some organ systems may be more prone to psychosomatic disorders. Heart, stomach, the skin, joints, and connective tissue (collagen) are the easily affected parts.

Angina, irregular heartbeats, chest pain, asthma, headache, migraine, high blood pressure, inflammatory bowel diseases like irritable bowel syndrome, Crohn's disease, chronic ulcerative colitis, thyrotoxicosis eczema, obesity, arthritis, peptic ulcers syncope and urticaria are a few of the innumerable psychosomatic disorders.

Treatment

A combined approach by the psychiatrist and the physician or surgeon treating the (patient)is desirable. The psychiatrist allows the sufferer to ventilate his fears. Group therapy, family network therapy, behavioral therapy and use of anxiolytic, antipsychotic or antidepressant medicines which suit the individual patient can be given. Parallel therapies like exercise, yoga, pranayam and meditation also play a useful role.

HIV and AIDS

Neuropsychiatric aspects

The names HIV and AIDs are common knowledge these days though knowledge about them is not detailed and many of their aspects are not known.

AIDS means,'Acquired Immunodeficiency Syndrome' and HIV means,'Human immunodeficiency virus'. HIV is transmitted through bodily fluids such as blood, vaginal secretions and semen. A common mode is transmission through unsafe sex, but it can also come through use of needles and syringes during blood transfusion, and can be passed from the mother to foetus too.

Half knowledge about HIV and AIDs, or even apprehension of infection can lead to psychiatric problems. There are of course many more neuropsychiatric problems of actual infection. Mental disorders seen in HIV patients are dementia, mood disorders and personality changes due to the medical condition. Depression, acute psychosis and mania are frequently seen in these patients. The central nervous system can be affected by HIV. Even before other signs are exhibited, 60% of people exhibit neurological symptoms. Brain involvement is seen in the post mortem (autopsy) of 75 to 90 % patients who die because of HIV-AIDS.

Treatment

Prevention by safe sex is the best bet. Anti-HIV medications from an expert physician and monitoring of the viral counts, prevention of opportunistic infection can help to some extent. Psychiatric help for the neuro psychiatric part is valuable.

Secondary Headache

A brain abscess can have its source in the ear, teeth, paranasal air sinuses or remote organs like lungs, heart and kidney. It could also be because of skull fracture, splinters and bullets.

Secondary headaches are called secondary because the cause is some primary disease but by no means are they of secondary importance. In fact they must be given immediate and detailed attention, evaluation and prompt treatment of the root cause.

The primary causes can be

1) Meningeal inflammations – encephalitis (viral) or meningitis (bacterial)

2) Bleeding in and around the brain.

3) Brain tumors - benign and malignant.

4) Inflammatory diseases of arteries and veins of the brain.

5) Acute closed angle glaucoma.

Meningitis – Encephalitis

Meninges of the brain are the protective clothing of the brain taking all the brunt of infections due to viruses and bacteria. These infections are rare as compared to other organs.

The causes of Encephalitis are viral infections of the meninges.

Viral infections at other places in the body, enterovirus, influenza, herpes simplex, measles, mumps, rubella and rabies can travel to the meninges at times.

The symptoms of this disease are sudden fever, headache, vomiting, weakness, sensitivity to light (photophobia), confusion or irritability, drowsiness, unsteady gait and loss of balance. In severe cases loss of consciousness, epileptic fits and muscle paralysis occur which are bad omen. The frequent victims are children, the elderly and those whose immunity is lowered. The patient needs hospitalization for supportive nutrition and breathing assistance until recovery. There are very few effective medicines for these viruses. The chances of survival depend on the severity of infection. Sometimes some neurological defect is left among the survivors after recovery.

Ominous - Ascendence or G.B. Syndrome

Everybody likes to have an ascending curve in life, in learning, financial growth, physical growth and healthy life. However, we do not want growth in bad things. Gullain – Barre Syndrome (G.B. Syndrome) is one thing in which we certainly hate ascendance.

G. B. Syndrome

G. B. Syndrome is an acute polyneuropathy a disorder involving multiple peripheral nerves. Weakness of the muscles of the lower limbs is the starting point. There is a deep aching pain in the weakened muscles often comparable to the pain felt due to over-exercise. There is some loss of sensation, particularly loss of sense of position. There may be a mild loss of temperature sensation. The pains are self-limited and there is relief when mild pain killer medication is given. The urinary bladder sensation may be lost for a while in severe cases. There may be fluctuations in blood pressure. Fall in the B.P. on rising or standing up may be significant and can lead to collapsing or falling down.

The muscle weakness and later paralysis that starts in the lower limbs may start ascending in hours or days to muscles of the arms and face. If the lower cranial nerves are affected leading to bulbar (brain stem) weakness, it leads to difficulty in swallowing and maintaining respiration. All these patients must be hospitalized the moment this syndrome is detected. About one- third of these patients need ventilator support for tiding over the crisis. In severe cases, there may also be increase or irregularity of heart beats.

After carefully checking the history and clinical examination, examination of the CSF by lumbar puncture and electromyography (EMG) must be done.

Causes

Some infectious agents like viruses elicit an auto-immune response in the body. The antigens in the infective agent make the immune system of the body misinterpret and target its own nerves. The myelin (Lipid) sheath of the nerves is thus destroyed by the immune system which leads to the paralysis of the muscles.

Fortunately, it is a self-limiting disease. If proper supportive and ventilator assistance is provided, most of the patients recover over a period of time.

Bacterial Meningitis

Bacterial infections of the meninges are commonly caused by menigococci and pneumococci. 10% to 15% of the patients die of these infections, many a times within 24 hours. Those who survive are likely to be left with serious neurological defects.

The infection can spread to near ones (within 3-4 feet) with prolonged contact, through air borne droplets. Early and aggressive treatment with antibiotics is vital. Prevention by vaccination in early childhood is advisable. Fever, headache, neck stiffness and vomiting are salient features.

TB – Meningitis

This is the most common form of tubercular infection of the nervous system. Fever and headache are cardinal features in the beginning. Examination of the cerebro spinal fluid (CSF) by lumbar puncture is a useful diagnostic test. C. T. and MRI may show changes which are suggestive of this infection. Bacterial diagnosis takes a couple of weeks but one cannot wait that long. The anti-tubercular medications should be started without waiting for the bacterial confirmation.

About one third of these patients develop blockage in the circulation of the C.S.F. leading to hydrocephalus. If it does, it may need a bypass surgery of ventricular shunt.

Cavernous Sinus Thrombosis

This is a rare complication following infection of the face, sinus, teeth, eyes and ears. This infection leads to a clot formation (thrombosis) in the cavernous venous sinus underneath the brain and behind the eye sockets. The death rate in this condition is very high (30-50%).

The symptoms are severe headache, swelling, redness, irritation around one or both eyes, drooping eyelids, inability to move the eyeballs, high fever and loss of vision or double vision. Sometimes there is pain and numbness around eyes or face, fatigue and epileptic fits.

Formation of a blood clot in the cavernous sinus by the immune system leads to prevention or spread of the infection. However, the clot raises the pressure inside the brain and this increased pressure can lead to damage to the brain and, finally, death. C.T and MRI scans are very handy in the diagnosis. Examination of blood and the CSF test for infection is an additional help in diagnosis.

Treatment

High doses of antibiotics given through intravenous route, steroids and blood thinners are additional help to tide over. If the patient does not respond to medical treatment, surgery to drain fluid can be lifesaving.

Brain Abscess

Brain abscess causes damage in two ways. As the cranium is a very tight compartment with no space for any alien substance, the abscess increases the intracranial pressure. It also produces symptoms because of pressure on the neighboring, important brain centers and brain stem compression and this can cause hydrocephalus.

Symptoms

Brain abscess produces fever and constitutional symptoms like fatigue because of the infective element. Severe headache, vomiting, confusion, focal neurological symptoms like difficulty in speech, hemiparesis, drowsiness, confusion, epileptic fits or seizures and coma may occur because of its space occupying nature. Neurological examination, C.T. and MRI scans help in the diagnosis. Examination of the CSF by lumbar puncture is also useful.

The brain abscess is normally secondary to some other source of infection. Both need to be treated in order to prevent recurrence.

Treatment

It can be treated by giving appropriate antibiotics, reducing the intracranial pressure and draining the abscess at the earliest. If the treatment is started before coma sets in, mortality can be restricted to 5-20%, otherwise it is very high.

Brain Tumors – (Sol – Space Occupying Lesion)

A tumour is an abnormal growth of cells. It can be benign i. e. non-cancerous or cancerous. A tumour arising from any cell in the brain or spinal cord (neurones, glial and ependymal cells), the meninges, the blood vessels, lymphatic tissue, cranial nerves, pituitary gland and pineal gland are all grouped together as brain tumors. The cranium is packed house there is no room for foreign substances of any sort.

Tumours can be primarily developed in the nervous system or they might have come from some other part of the body.

Primary tumors in children are usually in the posterior (region) of the brain. In adults they are normally found in the anterior (front) two-thirds of the cerebral hemispheres, although they can occur in any part at any age. Brain tumors are more troublesome because of the pressure they exert in a tight space. There are two kinds of effects; one because of the increased intracranial pressure for want of space and the other producing localized symptoms because of the pressure exerted on part of normal brain invaded by the tumor. The site of the tumor can be found out by the localizing signs and symptoms produced and of course with CT and MRI scans.

Signs and Symptoms

They are as follows: headache, vomiting, altered state of consciousness, dilatation of the pupil and papilledema (prominent optic disc on fundoscopy) on the side of the tumour. If the tumour is obstructing the circulationof the CSF it produces symptoms of increased intracranial pressure sooner. This can easily lead to a lethal brain stem compression (coning of the brain stem).

Treatment

Prompt diagnosis and surgery are a must. If the tumour is not easily accessible for surgery, some collateral damage to healthy brain tissues might have to be accepted.

Swollen Headed

When success goes to the head of a person, he is called swollen headed. When injury leads to a swollen head, it is equally or more ominous. Let us consider the head injuries from a trivial trauma to a severe one.

Anything hitting the scalp whether blunt or sharp, can lead to a cut in the scalp. The scalp bleeds and continues to bleed longer than other cuts on the skin because the blood vessels of the scalp cannot retract easily. Applying pressure for a long time or suturing the cut is the way to stop the bleeding quickly. Nature knows that the brain is the most important of all organs in the body and, hence, has provided a very hard and rigid cranium, the clothing of the dura (tough coat), the arachnoid (shirt) and the pia (banian). In addition, the cerebro spinal fluid in between arachnoid and piamater provides buffering action and nutrition. The brain is provided with a rich network of blood vessels considering the higher need for oxygen and glucose (20% of the total body needs).

If the trauma is very severe, the cranial bones can get fractured and this leads to bleeding between the bone and the dura (extradural hematoma), bleeding between the dura and arachoid (the subdural hematoma) or bleeding deeper than the arachnoid (sub arachnoid hemorrhage). All of them are dangerous and need prompt treatment. When there is a tear in the dura with a facture to the skullbone the CSF leaks through the wound or through the nose or ear if the fracture involves the base of the skull along with dural tear. This increases the chances of infection. High velocity objects like bullets or splinters after explosions can drive pieces of bone or foreign objects deep into the brain substance. They are dangerous lead to bleeding, infection, damage to the brain substance and are likely to be fatal. All foreign material must be removed surgically at the earliest. All hematomas need to be drained. A good antibiotic cover and life support system should be in place promptly.

Head Injuries

All injuries to scalp, skull or brain are termed as head injuries. The injury can damage neurological tissues of brain or nerves. It can cause bleeding at different depths. At times there may not be a fracture, hematoma or neuronal injury but the brain may be shaken very vigorously inside the skull. This also leads to temporary unconsciousness and some swelling of the brain. This is called cerebral concussion.

All head injuries must be observed in a hospital for 24-48 hours. Sometimes signs and symptom appear after few hours and progress rapidly (subdural or extramural haematoma), at times there is a delayed (gradual) ooze which comes out from venous blood. It may take days or weeks to manifest.

Signs and Symptoms

The signs and symptoms to watch for are: drowsiness, confusion, behavioral abnormality, loss of consciousness, headache, vomiting and mismatched pupils of the eye. There may be localizing signs if there is a neuronal injury or a haematoma pressing on the brain tissues. There may be bleeding or CSF may flow from nose or ears.

After checking the history of the injury and neurological examination, CT or MRI scans may give fair amount of information on the damage.

The depressed fracture of the skull bone compressing the brain, the hematomas pressing on the brain and splinter injuries of all sorts need urgent surgical measures. Even in the absence of these, there could be brain edema (swollen brain) which needs prompt medical and if need be surgical measures to reduce brain damage because the rigid cranial bones cannot provide space for the swollen brain.

Countrecoup Injury

At times the object hits one side and the part on the opposite side of the brain shows injury. This is because the brain is pushed to the opposite side in the cranial vault, brushing it crushing the inside of the skull and getting damaged. This type of injury is called countrecoup injury. This may be in the form of a hematoma or laceration of the brain substance.

It is common knowledge that parts of the brain control opposite sides of the body. This is the reason why injury to the right side of brain will affect left side of body and vice-versa.

Milder or repetitive (boxing) injuries can lead to dementia (forgetfulness) or Alzheimers in later life, but severe injuries can lead to coma or death.

BEWARE OF A SWOLLEN HEAD IRRESPECTIVE OF THE CAUSE.

19 Brain on Strike

Striking work is a commonly used tool by the working class in the present industrialised society, of late the officers have also resorted to go on strike. Has any body heard that the owner of the organisation going on strike?

It is rare, but can happen in the most well organized and industrious human body. In the normal course all the organs and systems, the basic units of the body and the cells are working relentlessly, round the clock right from birth to death. There is a hierarchy of cells, tissues and organ systems. The master controller is the brain, which is the head of the organization and this brain can also go on strike, Partially!! Partially, because it will still try to continue the essential services in the body like breathing, circulation of blood, digestion and excretion of waste products. Doctors call it stroke. Why does it happen and when?

The brain has to work very hard, hence its need for fuel: glucose and oxygen is highest. About 20% of glucose and oxygen is needed for the hard and non-stop work the brain has to do. The brain is about 2% of the body weight but its need for energy is 20%. This shows how hard the brain has to work. This is the reason why the brain has a very rich blood supply.

The cause of stroke is the loss of blood supply to the brain. If for some reason the blood supply to a part of, or the entire brain is reduced even slightly the results are damaging. This can happen in two ways - either by blocking a blood vessel of a part of the brain partially by an atherosclerotic patch, an embolus (plaque, blood clot, fat, or septic embolus) or causing a block by a large embolus depriving the neurons (the brain cells) of blood leading to their death. The other factor that can lead to the same result is bleeding from a blood vessel compressing the brain substance or failing to carry the blood to its destination.

The process of narrowing of the blood vessels can be gradual because of atherosclerotic patches. These patches are more common in people with raised sugar levels, cholesterol and lipids in blood. In short patients of diabetes and high blood pressure are at higher risks because of both; blockage of arteries and bleeding from the arteries or blockage of the veins. Such risks increase with advancing age and obesity. Divorced persons are more prone to it if there is a history of stroke in the family. Stroke is defined as a neurological deficit of cerebrovascular cause that persists beyond 24 hours or results in death within 24 hours.

Carotid Artery Disease –

The Carotid Artery is the main artery that passes up through the neck to supply blood to each half of the brain. Carotid arteries become narrow because of atherosclerosis like any other artery in the body. This can lead to stroke (paralysis). The entire brain is very vulnerable to the lack of blood. It can sustain itself for a maximum of 4 minutes without blood supply. Carotid disease in the mild form is treated by using medication. More severe narrowing is treated by carotid stents, while using a filter protection device to prevent small clots and bits of plaque from traveling up and blocking smaller arteries in the brain. This stenting is done via the groin artery. Thus carotid artery stenting is an alternative to open surgical removal of the plaque. Arteries inside the skull may also need stenting if narrowed; but it is riskier compared to carotid angioplasty since small arteries are fragile and are likely to bleed easily.

Intra Cranial Aneurysms

Aneurysms are small balloons produced because of weaknesses in the part of the arterial wall, which   is likely to burst and bleed. Even a small aneurysm bleeding in the brain can be fatal. A specialized embolization procedure known as endovascular coiling is required to stop this bleeding. These coils are very expensive but life saving.

AVMs

Arterio Venous Malformationsare of different types – Arterial, Arterio-venous, Venous and Capillary. These are most commonly seen in brain. If untreated, AVMs can rupture causing life threatening bleeding. Interventional radiologists can often treat this without surgery by guiding thin catheters to the affected part and injecting a substance (glue) that blocks the supply of blood to the affected blood vessels.

In the early stages of development, the embryo has a complex network of blood vessels which are being formed. There is no clear division in arteries, capillaries and veins. Later, a pattern starts developing. The vessels carrying blood from the heart and arteries develop an elastic coat and muscles in their walls. The arteries become progressively small in diameter as they show branching and re-branching. The smallest arteriole branches into smaller capillaries. These capillaries then lead to another set of capillaries which will carry blood from the tissues to smaller veins and then to larger veins and ultimately to the right auricle of the heart through the larger vene cavae. The muscle coat in the walls of the veins is sparse while the elastic coat is absent.

If for some reason the elastic and muscle coat in an arterial wall is sparse at a spot or absent, it leads to ballooning of that particular part of the artery. This is known as the aneurysm. Such an aneurysm in a branch of the artery in the brain can burst because of the higher pressure of blood in the arterial system. This is one of the causes of catastrophic cerebrovascular accidents leading to acute strokes. Similarly when the capillaries on the arterial side join the capillaries of the venous side without the inter-position of some normal tissues, it carries blood with higher pressure to the venous system. The venous system tries to adapt to the high pressure system by strengthening its muscle coat, but when it cannot sustain the pressure it starts dilating and becomes tortuous (Varicose). This is known as an arteriovenous malformation or AVM. Such AVMs are likely to burst leading to an acute cerebrovascular accident again.

Fortunately both of these malformations are exceptions rather than a rule. We have discussed brain strokes resulting from ischemia caused by an embolus or a thrombus earlier.

In this part I want to discuss a personal experience of a neuro-anatomist specialized in the study of the structure of the brain, Jill Bolte Taylor from the U.S.

Until the age of 37, Jill was leading normal life, working as a neuro-anatomist. She was doing research on the brain, teaching and campaigning for the cause of donating the brain after death for research purposes. On 10th December 1996 she experienced a massive stroke when a blood vessel from AVM in the left side of her brain suddenly exploded. She was not aware of any AVM in her brain till that moment.

A brain scientist that she was, she observed her mind completely deteriorate to the point that she could not walk, talk, read, write, or recall anything of her life all within the space of four hours. As the left side of the brain was damaged, the rational detail-and time-oriented side swung in and out of function. Taylor alternated between two distinct and opposite realities. The euphoric nirvana of the intuitive and kinesthetic right brain in which she felt a sense of complete well-being and peace; and the logical, sequential left brain which recognized Jill was having a stroke and enabled her to seek help before she was lost completely.

It took eight long years for her to completely recover.

Today Taylor is convinced that the stroke was the best thing that could have happened to her. It has taught her that the feeling of nirvana is never more than a mere thought away. By stepping to the right side of our brain, we can all uncover the feelings of well-being and peace that are so often sidelined by our brain chatter.

She calls this experience - "My stroke of insight".

With due respect to Jill, I beg to differ on certain statements made by her. The first and foremost is about remembering vividly the details of incidents that happened eight years after the traumatizing experience of stroke. This is incomprehensible. The other important thing is, how can any human being on earth suffering from sharp throbbing pain behind right eye, irritated and bewildered from the sixth minute of onset of the stroke feel peaceful and euphoric Nirvana at the same time? And if this is true, why did she try to come out of this divine state to the stark practical realities of life.

But the readers were impressed. I think the reader is impressed if he reads anything in the form of a printed book, especially if it is written by a doctor. I think we should be rational and should take these statements with a pinch of salt. We should be analytical and scientific.

All of these vascular causes will ultimately lead to the reduction of the flow of blood to part of the brain and death of the neurons in the area to be supplied. People who indulge in consumption of excess alcohol and tobacco in any form are at much higher risk of cerebrovascular accident. Another group having problems like aneurysm and Arterio Venous Malformation (AVM). The risk of bleeding from these anomalies subjects these people to much higher risks of Cerebro Vascular Accident(C.V.A).

A small percentage of sufferers get some warning signals in the form of Transient Ischemic Attacks(T. I. A).This may be due to a temporary spasm of the artery or due to a small embolus getting dislodged soon. Some of the signs and symptoms are common irrespective of the causative factor while some are specific to the cause and to the area of the brain that is affected.

There may be loss of smell, taste, hearing or vision (total or partial) decreased gag reflex (swallowing sensation), pupillary reflexes, drooping of eyelids and decreased breathing or reduced heart rate.

Small strokes may not cause symptoms but can still damage brain tissue.

Brain stroke is a medical emergency. It needs to be attended to promptly.

Clinical examination, record of blood pressure, examination of blood for sugar cholesterol and amino acids are to be done first. Sonography, Colour Doppler test of the carotid (neck) arteries to look for narrowing, clots and carotid angiography should follow.

C.T. and MRI scans of the brain with angiography, echocardiography of the heart to look for blood clots or vegetations in the heart all need to be done promptly.

The primary goal of treating ischemic stroke is to restore flow of blood to the brain. A Tissue Plasminogen Activator (TPA) is injected in the vein of the arm. At times of angioplasty putting a stent after balloon dilatation to keep the blood flow going is needed.

If the stroke is because of bleeding due to aneurysm, the clipping or embolisation of the aneurysm is done. Arterio-venous malformation needs open surgery whenever it can be accessed. Most stroke victims need rehabilitation in the form of speech therapy, occupational therapy and physical therapy. Involvement of the family in these therapies is crucial. Use of stem cell therapy for strokes is being researched.

Prevention

Prevention is always better than cure. This can be achieved by keeping blood sugar and cholesterol under control. It is advisable to totally stop tobacco consumption in any form, reduce sugar, fat and sodium intake in the diet, keep alcohol consumption to a minimum or observe complete abstinence. Stress levels should be kept down with the help of moderate physical exercise, yoga, pranayam and meditation. One study about diet has drawn a conclusion that consumption of tomatoes and a mediterranean diet helps prevent the genetic risk of a stroke.

Emotional Changes after a Stroke

If one is lucky to survive a brain stroke many times he has a changed personality. This is because of the hypoxic damage to part of the brain. These people have mood swings or

Within a few seconds or minutes of having a stroke the brain cells begin to die and symptoms begin to show. The common symptoms are trouble in walking, loss of balance and co-ordination, difficulty in speech, dizziness numbness, weakness or paralysis, blurred, blackened or double vision, sudden severe headache and confusion.

uncontrollable emotions for no reason e.g. crying or laughing for no reason. They may have depression, anxiety, irritability or apathy. All these are due to damage of the area in the brain that controls these functions. Another common behavioral change can be loss of normal inhibition. These people will do or say things that are socially inappropriate. They can be aggressive for no reason – verbally or physically. There may be seen a cognitive inability in thinking; for instance, difficulty in solving problems. They can have dementia (loss of memory) and other memory problems.

These patients need caring relatives or friends and the help of a physician as well as a psychiatrist.

Some people are also transformed after a brain stroke. They tend to be more philosophical and believers in God, in the life after death and rebirth.

Experimental studies on Tibetan monks using f-MRI-shows that with meditation they are able to minimize activity in the left side of the brain and increase the activity of the right side. This results in philosophical behavior, firm faith in Nirvana, life after death and rebirth. This is the effect achieved by shutting the logical rational role of the left side.

20 Evolution And History of Religions

The earth was born more than 4.5 billion years ago with no life on it. The conditions on the earth were not conducive for creation or survival of life in any form. Life started here by a chance chemical reaction in the minutest form first in the sea. Gradually the unicellular, then multicellular plant and organisms developed in the seas. The aquatic animals grew in size and form. Some of them started to crawl on the land; we know them as amphibians. Further evolutionary processes led to plants, trees, animals birds and ultimately to highly evolved and intelligent human beings. So life started in the minutest form millions of years from now. In this chain of life, human beings are the youngest, may be 1- 2 lakh years old.

Gods were created by human beings not more than 8000 or 10000 years ago. Gods assumed different forms and names in different geographical areas. The leaders in the tribes were god's men. They laid down certain ethical principles for human beings to follow. These were given names of religion. Religions were also bound to vary according to the different forms of gods in different geographical areas. As the means of communication increased, different tribes discovered each other. The initial reaction was that of fear and confrontation. There was no common language of communication. Any new tribe was thought to be hostile. There used to be competition for earthly belongings, whether food or cattle, water or land. Gradually, the believers of one god and one religion were united on the basis of that god and religious principles and together they fought with people of other faiths and gods.

See the irony! A large section of educated or so-called civilized societies still believe in their own religion and criticize that of others. One thing common in most of the religions is that the God is almighty. He created the universe and nothing on the earth can happen without his knowledge concurrence and desire.

I wonder whether most of us have forgotten that the human race is only 1-2 lakh years old and the animal and plant kingdom is 20-30 crore years old. God is a concept created by the youngest of the animals, man, only 8-10 thousand years ago. God is not seen by anybody. But if He is the Creator, why would he want to see plants, animals and human beings suffer for basic things like pure air, water, shelter etc? Why do we have a food chain in which one needs to kill one to satisfy the hunger of the other? Why could food not be created by the Almighty separately like air and water? Perhaps, all the religious leaders will frown at me if they read what I am writing or kill me to stop my propagation of such thoughts. I have tried to read, discuss and argue with people about God, different faiths and the ultimate of religious practices and acts but could not be satisfied.

Men Of God

As I cannot see god it becomes difficult for me to believe in the existence or concept of god. I think seeing is believing, but I would

It is an unfortunate fact that a large number of lives were lost in these so-called religious wars and they outnumber loss of life due to other causes. The teachings of all the religions are good. Most of them advocate love and condemn hatred and enmity, but still more wars were fought and are fought in the name of religion even in today's so-called civilized society. not under-estimate or criticize those who are believers.

A few god-men in almost all religions preach good things, and teach respect for other religions. In fact, many clerics try to impress how their own religion is supreme. However some of them advise us to be selfless, to be devoted to God and try to please Him by offering prayers and leading a pious life and spending maximum possible time for these activities. They advise us to be altruistic and to sacrifice most of the worldly pleasures. Some religions even go further by advising to torture your own body by fasting and in many other ways. They believe in rebirth. Their teaching is that your soul is immortal; it keeps changing the body like we change our clothes. It may be in human or any other form depending on the good or bad deeds done in this birth. Especially Jainism, Buddhism and Hinduism advocate the way of suffering as a sure shot for getting to "MOKSHA" or "NIRVANA". The rebirth theory says you will get human life again only by doing a lot of good deeds in this life. But the ultimate aim of the soul should be to get out of this birth cycle.

Moksha

Moksha is also called ViMoksha, Mukti, Vimukti, Nirvana and by many other names in philosophy. It means the liberation of human beings from the cycle of birth and death to a state of knowledge, peace and bliss. I do not know whether it applies to other life forms; from unicellular life forms to elephants and from planktons to huge trees. There are many ways suggested to human beings for attaining Moksha. The other life forms have to do good deeds, (Punya) to come to the human form first and Moksha can be an option for them only after human form. I fail to understand how these poor and often helpless life forms can attempt good deeds to earn punya. Islam calls it Jannat Christians heaven Hindus call it swarg and so on. People with different religious faiths differ in their concepts of God and good deeds. But all of them believe in the death and birth cycle. They have concepts like Avidya (Ignorance) of human beings about the universe or the ultimate principle, the ultimate knowledge about the soul and oneness of the largest soul (The GOD). The aim is to sacrifice the physical body and attain freedom, self realization and self knowledge about the oneness of the universe in the nonphysical or metaphysical form. However, all the religious philosophies have their own concepts of the means to achieve liberation. Philosophers in the same religion also differ widely in their thinking and practices. Starting from selflessness, altruism, yoga, meditation, Japa (reciting Gods names repeatedly), endurance, sacrificing worldly pleasures and accepting suffering or Atma klesha to embracing death voluntarily(Samadhi). On the other hand many ways of going into a trance have been suggested from dancing and singing with a rhythm to having sexual orgasms. Some people resort to drugs such as opium, L.S.D. and anesthetic agents like ketamine to achieve trance. All of these are means of attaining peace – divine or human.

Some philosophies advocate remaining in samsara (routine human life). They advise to follow four Purusharthas (Ethics) a) Dharma (virtuous proper moral life) b)Artha (material prosperity, income, security as means of life) c)Kama (pleasure, sensuality, emotional, fulfilment)which are the three goals of life and the fourth is Moksha as described above.

The four stages of human life have been described in Hindu shastras as:

1) Bramhacharyashram- studentship and remaining bachelor

2) Gruhasthashram – getting married earning bread for the family and shouldering all the family responsibilities

3) Vanaprasthashram – retired life spent with the spouse

4) Sanyashashram- spending time in isolation away from the society.

If you follow all of these honestly, you have fulfilled your life's duty. You can resort to religious practices in all ashrams more so in the last lap. However, this may not be sufficient to attain Moksha. If you have not taken special efforts to attain enlightenment.

Ways and Means of Attaining Moksha

The definition and meaning of Moksha differs from scholar to scholar. Moksha is liberation, but from what and how is a hotly debated question amongst the wise and learned men. This is bound to happen because the discussion is about a nonphysical entity. It is about concepts. No two minds on earth can think alike. When there is a difference of opinions on the definition and meaning there is bound to be a difference in the ways and means to achieve Moksha. There will be no common laws to follow.

In spite of all these differences there is a general congruity among these people that attaining Moksha means jivan-mukti (liberation) from present life (body) and Videha-mukti (incorporeal emancipation) is the freedom from any corporeal state (physical body) hereafter. After Videha-mukti you are a part of the universal soul. You cease to exist as you or me. Everything is one; the larger soul - GOD. You are a part of Him.

Once we accept that there is a single, universal soul, then the idea of incarnations of God sounds funny. In mythologies of many religions, it is believed that God is born on the earth in human form and brings solace to the human race whenever it is in difficulty because of bad elements on the earth. Does this mean that God who takes human form on the earth has not achieved Videha-mukti?

If a human being has to die to be enlightened. If the ultimate goal in life is to get the torch of enlightenment, then why strive to do anything else? If the easiest way to get knowledge is to meditate to recite names of God then why on earth should man learn anything else at all? Are all those human beings who learn various subjects or do research to demystify the laws and principles of nature crazy?

Transcendence

The soul or spirit which is not seen, felt or perceived in any way is the concept of God created by man.

However, we hear of some metaphysical experiences narrated by persons who are near death. It may be a person having a severe heart attack, a severe trauma to the brain due to a physical accident, a cerebrovascular accident, anesthetic accident or some other health problem. There are many things common among the experiences narrated by different people suffering from these conditions all over the world. They talk about detachment from the body or out of body experiences, going through a dark tunnel and seeing bright light at the end of the tunnel, complete peace of mind, crossing a boundary and reaching the gods and departed souls of near and dear ones in the heaven. They have a conviction that they have actually experienced it. They come back with a changed philosophy of life like religious people. Children do not talk about God or souls if they have not known about it. This indicates the element of enculturation.

Exactly similar experiences are narrated by people who consume drugs like L.S.D. and Ketamine or patients having a tumor in the left temporal lobe of the brain.

Scientists are studying the brains of monks who can voluntarily achieve such state of mind.

Many science fiction films of yesteryears have been proved to be a reality now. Recently a science fiction film on transcendence has been released. This film is directed by Wall Pfister and the story has been written by Jack Pagen. The film is about Dr. Will Caster, a scientist motivated by curiosity about the nature of the universe. The scientists are working on a computer which should be responsive to human consciousness. Scientists believe that this will create technological transcendence. This is an attempt similar to building an intelligent and cognitive machine. Dr. Will is attacked by terrorists who believe in revolutionary independence from technology. Will's wife connects Will's likeness which survives his body's death to the internet so as to grow in capability and knowledge as per the desire expressed by Will before death.

Transcendence is attainment of the metaphysical state by a human being while he has physical existence. This concept of being a part of the universal oneness after leaving the physical body and having no state is called videha-mukti.

Thus Will's intelligence survives in the form of an intelligent, conscious computer. Ultimately, the terrorists destroy the intelligent machine using a virus and the dark era of the world without technologies dawns.

Neuroscientists and computer scientists are working together to decode the brain waves. The men of God, especially the Tibetan Buddhist Monks have developed and practiced techniques of meditation to derive physical and psychological benefits. Those who are dedicated to these techniques in a disciplined way can tap into the human organism's natural and biological systems to enable themselves with impressive capabilities. The metabolism of the body is reduced by 10-15% during sleep. But these accomplished monks can bring it down by 50%. Some of the monks can levitate and jump or glide to impressive distances. Some of the monks can raise the temperature of part of their body by nearly 200 while maintaining the internal temperature in the rest of the body at normal.

People who practice meditation get dissolution of thoughts in internal awareness of pure consciousness without objectification and merge in infinity.

Matthieu Ricard, a 66 year old Tibetan Monk and geneticist produced brain gamma waves linked to consciousness, attention, learning and memory which had never been recorded by neuroscientists. This is the secret of his success in achieving bliss.

He claims that meditating is like exercising the mind. Anybody can be happy or blissful by simply training his own brain. Ricard demonstrated excessive activity in the right side of his brain. This practice or exercise has given him a capacity for happiness and has reduced propensity for negativity. He says this is the science of the mind. David Lynch explains that consciousness, creativity and benefits of Transcendental Meditation (T.M.) can affect creativity and overall learning and expansion of the human mind.

21 To Heaven and Back

Near Death Experiences (NDE)

NDE is a strange experience which brings about a feeling of detachment from the body, and causes powerful hallucinations, some of the notable ones being a tunnel experience, a bright light, and God and the souls of our loved ones who have departed for heaven. This usually occurs when accidental trauma or cardiac arrest deprives the brain of oxygen. Lack of sleep over a long period of time can also lead to euphoria and end in irritability or hallucinations. High fever leads to irritability and a strange impression which we call delirium. The aura felt by epileptics just before a seizure is caused by excessive neural activity in the brain. If it starts in the temporal lobe, it may produce transcendent feelings often similar to those felt during peak experiences.

People all over the world have different conceptions of God, heaven, hell, the soul, rebirth, and life after death. Some concepts differ with religion and faith, whereas others are overlapping. But each and every one of them has something in common - All good things are pertaining to heaven. I am sure nobody with such faith would prefer The earth over living with his chosen God and the souls of his ancestors.

We often hear about people who have narrowly escaped death and had a heavenly experience. These experiences are called Near Death Experiences (NDE). The earliest account of a NDE can be traced back to 4th century B.C. At present, a lot of research and analysis is taking place with regards to that account. In 1968, Celia Green published an analysis of 400 firsthand experiences of Near Death Experiences. Before this point in history, they were termed as perceptual experiences or hallucinations. Further interest was sparked in the subject by John Weiss in 1972 and Raymand Moody in 1975. Thornard (2013) said NDE cannot be considered as an example of an event in which person imagines memories. Physiological origins could lead them to be perceived, although not lived in reality.

Various Experiences

People near death often experience feelings of levitation, a fluid state, total serenity, security, warmth, detachment from the body, the presence of light, and the experience of absolute dissolution.

People who have experienced an NDE say that they saw their body from a distance. They say their soul was watching the efforts taken by the doctors and nurses in the resuscitation room. They say their souls passed to heaven, they met and talked to God and to the souls of their deceased relatives. They experienced the transcendence of their egotic and spaciotemporal boundaries.

The elements they describe tend to correspond with the cultural, philosophical and religious beliefs of the person experiencing the NDE. The Christians see Jesus, Buddhists see Buddha, and so on. This is absolute, except in the case of the Africans. The Africans believe rewards and punishments come to people during the course of their life itself. They do not believe in life after death or rebirth. In NDEs, many Africans narrate a tunnel experience, a sense of moving up or going through a dark passageway or even climbing a staircase, to see a sudden powerfully blinding light, and being swept over by an intense feeling of unconditional love or acceptance. Their life is reviewed, and they receive knowledge abut the life and nature of the universe. They get a feeling that they have approached a border, and make the decision to return to the earth and their body, often reluctantly.

Some of the factors leading to NDEs are cardiac arrest alongside a myocardial infarction or anaesthetic complication, shock due to severe blood loss, preoperative complications, septic or anaphylactic shock, electrocution or a coma due to trauma to the head, bleeding in the substance of the brain or infarction of the brain, attempted suicide, drowning, asphyxia, apnea and serious depression.

Most of the NDE sufferers have pleasant experiences pertaining to heaven, but about 1% lose their way and see hell instead of heaven. They experience a sensation of falling down, mourning and despair, even tormenting fire. They visit dark, distressing, desolate areas.

High fever leads to irritability and a strange experience which we call delirium. The aura felt by epileptics just before the seizure is caused by excessive neural activity. If it starts in temporal lobe it may produce transcendent feelings similar to those felt during peak experience.

People with depressing experiences were not marked by religious or suicidal backgrounds. The long term recall of NDEs was the same and did not change over time in both the groups.

Children have also been subject to NDEs. Very young children tend to report irrational experiences that have some common

NDE elements. As the children get older, their religious teachings often colour their NDEs with more spiritual connotations such as meeting God. In conclusion, what is embedded in the mind by enculturation is reaped in the NDE.

Some people who have experienced NDEs think of these experiences as a reprieve or 'second chance' before the end. I think it is possible that every dying person has to experience this. The only problem is that they do not survive to share what they felt. They have no return ticket from either heaven or hell.

The Logic

Cognitive neuroscience addresses the question of how physiological functions like human feelings and sensations are produced by neural circuitry (including the brain). Brain activity scans are not typically performed when the patient is being resuscitated. The topmost priority is to save the person's life rather than scan the brain for NDE. In animal experiments, heightened brain activity has been recorded In rats following cardiac arrest.

Dieguez (2008) and Olaf Blanke (2009) have published accounts presenting evidence on the brain based nature of near death experiences.

Parnia (2010) asserted on the basis of evidence that even after the process of death has started in a person, the mental and cognitive processes may continue for a set period of time. Even if the EEG is flat, there may still be brain activity that could be detected using a f-MRI, PET scan or CAT scan. He described the process of death as "essentially a global stroke of the brain." Hence, like any stroke process, one would not expect the entire mind or consciousness to be lost immediately.

Computational Psychology

Modelling of NDEs by S.L. Thaler in 1993 using artificial neural network has shown that many aspects of the core of NDEs can be achieved through simulated neuron death. In the course of such simulations, the essential features of the NDE such as life review, heaven, hell and out of body experiences etc. are observed. It is a generation of confabulations of false memories. Memories, whether related to direct experience or not, can be seeded upon arrays of such inactive brain cells.

NDEs are neither real experiences nor spiritual voyages, but a function of the dying brain. All brains regardless of where they are from in the world, die in the same way, that is, by Hypoxia. It is not because the dying person is journeying towards a beautiful afterlife, but because the neurotransmitters in the brain are shutting down and that process is creating the same lovely illusions for all who are near death. In short, NDEs are nothing more than a series of brain reactions.

It is a known fact that an anaesthetic drug, Ketamine can produce many features similar to that of NDEs, particularly, the out of body experience. It is possible that a ketamine like substance is released by the body at the time of the NDE. Dr. Ronald Siegel, a Professor of Psychology rejected the spiritual and mystical importance of NDEs. He reproduced NDEs in volunteers by giving them LSD. Some features of the NDE are known to occur in a type of epilepsy associated with damage to the temporal lobe of the brain. Researchers could replicate some elements of NDEs, such as leaving behind oneself, a sense of memories flashing past by electrically stimulating the temporal lobe, the stress of being near death, or thinking that one is near death, may in some way, cause the stimulation of this lobe. There is some evidence to support this theory when we see NDEs reported by people who suffer strokes which affect this part of the brain, or have tumors in this part of the brain.

Floating in air without wings (out of body experience)

This can also happen if one's right parietal lobe is stimulated with an electrode while one is still conscious and awake, he will momentarily feel that he is floating near the ceiling, watching his own body down below (NDE like experience). He has an out of body experience without any disease in a fully conscious state.

Jill Bolte Taylor, the author of the book, " My stroke of insight " had an AVM in the left temporal lobe and she showed some NDE like symptoms i.e. An out of body experience and a feeling of the fluid state, when she had bleeding from her AVM.

To summarise and pinpoint the genesis and veracity of NDEs would be being too simplistic. I have some personal views on the subject.

The human brain is the most evolved one of all the living beings on Earth. The basic function of the brain is to help an organism to survive, propagate and evolve. It is essential to make the organism aware of it's environment, to adapt to it, to procure food for its body and respond to the environment in a suitable manner. It also has to control digestion, excretion, circulation of the blood and respiration. All these basic tasks are performed by the brains of organisms even on the lower rung of the evolution ladder. All these functions are represented in the hind brain of human beings. In the process of evolution, the midbrain developed before the forebrain. The forebrain in humans is the largest part of the brain and has been given faculties for higher functions like speech, memory, thinking, imagination and intelligence. These distinguished faculties have given humans the highest status in the animal kingdom.

In case of life threatening situations, the highest priority of the brain is to preserve the basic vital functions of the body even at the cost of the highest and latest functions of the brain. This is the reason why the brain loses the faculties of speech, thinking and memory of the left brain before that of the right brain. The left brain is the part which deals with logical and practical thinking while the right brain cares more for human values and thinks about moral and religious values.

I believe that if this happens at the time of a NDE, there may be a change in the personality of the patient during and after the NDE, due to the involvement of the right brain. People after NDEs are convinced that they have been to heaven. Alcoholics turn sober. Hardened criminals try to be saintly. Atheists become believers. These people become more altruistic, less materialistic and more loving. They begin to feel that all people are good. In other words, we may say that these people become less practical, find it difficult to face everyday life, and lose ego boosting achievements.

In a study conducted in this respect, 21% of the people denied after effects of NDE, 19% claimed radical change as if they had become a different person, and the remaining 61% reported significant life changing thinking.

To conclude, hypoxia of the brain due to any reason leads to changes in the neurotransmitters in the brain. This produces global changes in the brain leading to various experiences of NDE. commensurate with age and enculturation of the individual. Those who survive the hypoxia live to tell about the experiences but majority of the people cannot live to tell us about it.

22 Science And Religion Meet

In India, we have a proverb,which translates to- "You cannot see heaven (and the gods) unless you die." This is not the truth any longer. Now you can see heaven in all it's glory without dying. A compilation of scientific data about near death experiences shows that people who had severe heart attacks, accidents with trauma to the brain, cerebro-vascular accidents (especially involving the left temporal lobe of the brain), fainting and unconsciousness following severe blood loss or shock all lead to near death experiences(NDE). The people who survive and regain consciousness narrate their out-of-body experiences as being in a fluid state, merging into the universe and a tunnel with a bright light at the end of it and then meeting their dear ones who had died earlier and of course their chosen gods (depending on the culture in which they have been brought up). Not only these but anaesthetic drugs like Ketamine and L.S.D. can give you these divine experiences without going near death or actually dying.

A normal conscious person has only heard of heaven and the gods. He has no experience or evidence. These are only blind beliefs, often unshakable under any circumstances.

The clerics or messengers of God often boast that the ultimate truth or religious faith begins where science ends. Does science really end anywhere? Can it stop it's progress at any point in time? No! There is no end to science. It is an ever ongoing process. Scientists do not discover anything new. All that goes up comes down. When Isaac Newton saw an apple fall down from a tree, he was the first person on the earth to analyze and talk about the force of gravity. Gravity did not start on that day. It existed from the time the Earth was created. It was only demystified by a human being for the first time. The same can be said about all the scientific discoveries to date. They are present in nature; some scientists have simply unveiled them for human beings. There are many more things in nature waiting to be discovered. This will always be an ongoing process. This is always unending. Science does not stop progressing. The process does not end at any time.

The men of God always talk about the ultimate truth, about self realization. What is it? Can it be proved? Is there any conclusive evidence of it all?

Before the advent of the logical scientific explanations based on evidence in the modern era, all the good events in nature were looked upon as the blessings of God by the common God-fearing human beings. They also interpreted natural disasters like earthquakes, volcanoes, tornados, tsunamis, floods and the ice age as the rage of the almighty in the heavens. As a matter of fact, all these were happening on a much larger scale and more frequently before the first signs of life on the earth. Man came much later and gods were created by man very recently.

We witnessed the disasters like the one in Kedarnath recently. Why would God kill thousands of his own devotees when they were only trying to please him by going on a pilgrimage? Why have people to guard the sacred homes of God, temples with sten guns and AK-47s, when the Gods themselves are Almighty? The irony is that the common God-fearing people do not utter a word even though they may be convinced that God's existence is questionable. They blame it all on the sins of their previous birth.

This is the result of deep rooted religious superstitions and the fear of the gods encultured for generations together. Things are gradually changing with education, scientific research and experiences. People, especially the younger generations are getting bolder, believing more in science than in the religious superstitions. This trend is gaining momentum. A beginning has been made but it will take quite some time for the common man to think rationally.

It has been said for a long time - Religion begins where science ends. The situation is now reversing. We are able to give scientific explanations for the concepts of transcendence, near death experiences like out-of-body experiences, levitation, the fluid state and the heavens and souls of the departed people by studying all the cases where blood supply is reduced to the left side of the brain, especially temporal lobe. We cannot risk a human life in an experiment to reduce blood supply to this part of brain and record observations. Another way is to study the brains of those who indulge in taking drugs like L.S.D., Ketamine etc which give such divine experiences to the people indulging in drug abuse.

It is often boasted by the clerics or the messengers of God that the ultimate truth or religious faith begins where science ends. Does science really end anywhere? Can it stop progress any time? No! There is no end to science. It is an ever ongoing process. Scientists do not discover anything new.

People with a tumor in the temporal lobe or epileptics (due to involvement of the temporal lobe)also report such divine experiences. This is where religious explanations come to an end and science emerges to give an explanation. Shall we say that Religion and Science meet here?

It is observed that with an increase in age, people become increasingly philosophical and religious. It is also a scientific fact that with an advance in age, the arteries of the whole body, including the brain, start narrowing. This in turn leads to decreased blood supply to the brain. Hence blood flow to the brain is said to reduce with increase in religiosity and philosophical change in behaviour.

To be simplistic, we can conclude that most of the revered religious achievements such as an out of the body experience, transcendence (moksha) and a feeling of bliss (ultimate knowledge and incomparable peace) can all be produced and achieved by various means such as meditation, breathing control, music or dance, drugs like LSD or Ketamine, temporal lobe epilepsy and lastly, a tumor, or reduced blood supply to the temporal lobe (whether voluntary or involuntary).

This can be experimented and proved like other science experiments.

Most of the mysteries relating to heaven or heavenly bodies have been deciphered by science by this method, and I am sure the rest will follow. Science will keep on progressing. There is no end to it, just as there is no end to the connection between science and religion.

Let us keep our minds open for a dialogue.

" This is not the end;

Let it be a new beginning."

Bibliography

We would like to thank the copyright owners for permitting to use the following images.

1.Wikipedia, the free encyclopedia, Material used under C R E A T I V E   C O M M O N S   P U B L I C   L I C E N S E (http://creativecommons.org/licenses/by-sa/3.0/)

a) http://en.m.wikipedia.org/wiki/Broca's_area

b) http://en.m.wikipedia.org/wiki/Anencephaly

c) http://en.m.wikipedia.org/wiki/Human_brain

2. WebMD: http://www.webmd.com/brain/picture-of-the-brain, ©2013, WebMD, LLC. All rights reserved

3. Image of Holo anencephaly, hydrocephalus, encephalocoele and menigocoee from Dr Sudhakar Jadhav and Dr Ravindra Vora of Paediatric Surgery Centre, Sangli.

www.ingramcontent.com/pod-product-compliance
Lightning Source LLC
Chambersburg PA
CBHW032348280326
41935CB00008B/491